Peter Alex

The Homeopathic Treatment of Lyme Disease

English Edition

Cover design by Ulrike Hirsch and Peter Alex
The black figure is an alchemic symbol for gold

Layout and production by Kara Adanalian: www.acmegfx.com

HomeopathyWest · 7829 Terrace Drive · El Cerrito, CA 94530 · USA
www.HomeopathyWest.com

First published 2005 as *Heilung Borreliosekranker mit Homoeopathie*

Printed on recycled paper
ISBN: 978-0-9754763-1-4

A percentage of the proceeds from the sale of this book go towards the restoration of Hahnemann's house in Torgau, Germany. This house is now the site of the Torgau International Homeopathic College.

Please visit www.hahnemann-torgau.de for more information on this project.

Torgau International Homeopathic College

Peter Alex

The Homeopathic Treatment of Lyme Disease

with contributions from: Bill Gray
Matthias Richter
Alize Timmerman
Frans Vermeulen
and others

English Edition
HomeopathyWest Publishing

Publisher's Note:

We are very pleased to present the English translation of Peter Alex's book on the homeopathic treatment of Lyme Disease, first published in German in 2005. The importance of this work cannot be overstated. In addition to the clarity of the author's presentation on the usefulness of Homeopathy in the treatment of Lyme disease, we also are gifted with his insight into the nature of epidemic disease, our positive interrelationship with bacteria and the trouble that may result whenever we disregard nature's laws. Written for the homeopath as well as the lay person interested in getting to the cause of illness, this booklet contains a wealth of philosophical information as well as cogent practical advice for the treatment of Lyme disease.

The internet is a good resource for finding a homeopath near you.
In the US and Canada, contact the National Center for Homeopathy:
http://nationalcenterforhomeopathy.org.

Other homeopathic practitioner directories can be found at:
www.homeopathicdirectory.com and www.wholehealthnow.com

Contents

Part 3

Translator's Preface

I first met Peter Alex in 2002, during the International Homeopathic Seminar, convened by Alize Timmerman in The Hague, Netherlands. We both had taken rooms at a hotel bordering Scheveningen beach, and at the end of a long day we had the opportunity to talk while watching the sun set on the ocean. Right away, I was impressed by Peter's sharp mind, his dedication to homeopathy, and also by his sense of fun.

Some months later Peter mailed me a copy of his just-published book on Lyme disease. At that point I recognized that if I were to comprehend a problem that greatly troubles people in northern Europe, I would have to blow the dust off my German dictionary, last thumbed years ago while delving into Faust as a student at the University of Toronto.

And it was well worth the effort. Peter, along with a phalanx of colleagues, has stepped into Samuel Hahnemann's big shoes, striving to stem an epidemic condition that threatens the well-being of their communities. Each year 250,000 people in Germany become infected with Lyme disease, while the number of undiagnosed cases cannot even be estimated. Employing homeopathic methods, Peter, together with his colleagues, has hit upon promising means both to cure the affliction, and also to prevent it from occurring in the first place. Obviously there are lessons here to learn for those across the pond, worried as they are about West Nile Virus and all the other beasts that may be slouching towards them.

Realizing that his book might fail to please anyone by attempting too much, Peter nevertheless risked addressing his *Heilung Borreliosekranker mit Homoeopathie* as much to the layperson as to the practitioner. But his gambit has succeeded wonderfully. Now in its second edition, there are more than 3,000 copies in circulation, making *Heilung* a homeopathic best-seller in Germany.

Centuries before Hahnemann, the Saxon people were defending their fertile land from foes large and small, from barbarians as well as bacteria. In doing so they accumulated a deep pool of sustaining knowledge. Today, in the midst of a Lyme epidemic, Peter seeks the source of the affliction in the trans-generational collective body, the place where miasms, or mass miseries, are stored. From this deep stratum pathology emanates. In this dark arena gentle homeopaths unsheathe their swords.

Peter identifies *Aurum arsenicosum* as the mineral substance which, in Saxony, best replicates the Lyme misery. Its bald mimicry can make the bully implode. In itself this represents a significant contribution to homeopathy. But Peter pursues the matter further, by proposing that Lyme disease has settled in as a miasm in his part of the world. No doubt Peter will be queried by his colleagues as to whether the Lyme complex actually warrants such a status. The term embodies a geopolitical dimension, to which not every rag-tag ailment can aspire. Sensing parallels with the life of Hahnemann, some critics may sniff that miasm-making is but a well-worn ploy on the part of a talented homeopath aspiring to an elite practice in Paris. It should be kept in mind, however, that a disease need only circulate in a population for several generations to entrench itself as a miasm. The critical variable is neither time nor space, but the degree of fit between the disease manifestation and the collective character of the population it besets.

Since our first meeting in The Hague, I have had several opportunities to visit Peter at his home in Saxony. He resides with his family only a few miles to the south of Torgau, where Samuel Hahnemann lived until 1811, one year after completing the first version of his *Organon*. After some archival research it was determined that Hahnemann's house still stands in sound condition in the centre of town. Currently it is undergoing extensive renovations. The loft has already been completely re-timbered. But the ground floor requires more exacting, tender care, since there are extensive Romanesque frescoes concealed beneath the drab plaster. We can imagine Hahnemann relaxing in his parlour, encircled by Attic deities bearing platters of viands and amphoras of wine. The *Internationales Homoeopathiekolleg Torgau*, which Peter chairs, is now housed on these venerable premises.

Though Peter has patiently proofed this text, I readily acknowledge any remaining errors as solely my own.

May each one of us in this brief lifetime encounter our mirror-like simillimum.

Douglas Smith, PhD, HD
Minden, Ontario, Canada

Acknowledgments

Nowadays, there is scarcely any technical publication, no matter how slim, that can claim sole authorship. There are always people who diligently gather material, sparing the author exhaustive labours, or who provide contributions, give helpful advice, and in the end correct the proofs. Since for various reasons not everyone is cited on the cover, the most important should be mentioned here with thanks — first of all, of course, to our patients, who time and again provide us with the chance to experience the potentials of our homeopathic method. Understandably their names will not be given here.

Thanks go to all the teachers of homeopathy, from whom I was able to learn and continue to learn. To name but a few: Ravi Roy, Manfred Tauscher, Dr. Rajan Sankaran and Dr. Jan Scholten.

Thanks are due my colleagues, with whom I maintain regular exchanges in order to examine my own work on a critical basis — and especially to those colleagues who contributed to the contents of this work: Alize Timmerman, Frans Vermeulen, Bill Gray, Matthias Richter, Rocco Kirch and Jens Kichner. Thanks also to my colleagues Drs. Amy Rothenberg and Paul Herscu, who permitted several cases to be cited from their *New England Journal of Homeopathic Medicine.*

For their thoughtful contributions to our discussion on the nature of matter, I especially wish to thank my colleagues Frans Vermeulen and Dr. Burghard Junghans.

Thanks are owed my collaborators Dr. Kostja Lazovsky, Antje Gredig and Susanne Koehn for the often tedious tasks that they took from my shoulders.

While reading this book you will enjoy the work of that most dedicated and skilled translator, the Canadian homeopath and astrologer, Douglas Smith, Ph.D., ND. It was a great pleasure to see him not only translate, but also re- structure the book and shape it according to the English reader's convenience. I am grateful for having been blessed with his help.

Thanks to Anneke Hogeland, the publisher of the English edition, who very spontaneously offered the service of her publishing house. Together with Judy Schriebman, they cared for the ends being tied together.

Last but not least my thanks goes to my family, who showed much understanding, when on account of various exigencies (as, for example, publications) our precious time together was cut short.

Recycled Paper

My activities for change in East Germany began in the late 1980's as a member of a group of environmentalists and later as a supporter of Greenpeace International. Seeing the forests in Europe dying due to acid rain profoundly shifted my consciousness. Travelling afterwards to Washington state in 1990 and seeing the huge clear cut areas there gave me a physical feeling of a red line having been crossed. This red line I feel is the limit for what mother earth can tolerate without being forced to throw us all off for the sake of maintenance of life on the planet. Since then, I see a big tree appearing behind every piece of virgin paper. Big trees deserve our awe and our listening to their thousands of years of history, instead of blowing our noses or wiping our behinds with them. So it goes without saying that I only use recycled paper everywhere, both in my household and in my office. And when I started writing articles for magazines or for books, I urged the editors and publishers to use recycled paper for the printing. It does not cost more than virgin paper in most countries, and it is a simple way of getting the message of the trees through to the readers, a message that otherwise is still too often overlooked.

—Peter Alex

Introduction

Apart from my veterinary studies, where Lyme disease played a minor role, I started getting interested in this phenomenon only in the late 1990's. Having since taken up treating humans, I found more and more clients reporting that they had tested positive for *borrelia*. I simply noted the first cases without making too much of it.

But soon enough, those who visited my office began pressing me with questions about tick bites and Lyme disease. Since it was tedious to answer the same questions hundreds of times over, I put together some leaflets addressing the questions most frequently asked. These I provided to anyone interested. Because of the great interest expressed, I sent one of these leaflets to the popular journal *Nature & Healing*. There I mentioned that I had begun collecting material towards eventual publication. I had in mind a period of several years, for I wanted to gather further observations and experiences in the treatment of a wide range of patients. Yet I didn't count on the strong response to my article. Within a few weeks I received more than 300 orders for my "publications." Many sufferers, but also medical doctors and naturopaths, requested that I send them my progress report. Fortunately, in 2003 I had colleagues who were prepared to place their cured cases at my disposal for publication, and my associate, Dr. Egon Krannich, published the resulting German volume. So we were able to satisfy these requests in that very same year.

Since the interest kept up unabated, this limited printing was eventually exhausted. Requests were made for a new edition. Thanks to the lively exchange, which the appearance of the "collation" unleashed, I was spurred on to further research. A number of cured cases emerged, which two years previous could not have been described as such. Also, we dedicated ourselves to the proving of new homeopathic remedies.

It was not by accident that I met Frans Vermeulen in June of 2004. He is one of the most knowledgeable scholars in the field of homeopathic Materia Medica. Nor was it by accident that his lecture topic was "Bacteria in General and Spirochetes in Particular." On this subject the two of us held a lively discussion. The fruits of this discussion have influenced this new edition every bit as much as further material from the literature.

As ever, to the standard question, "What do you advise, if I am diagnosed with Lyme disease?" I would give a standard reply: "As soon as possible seek out an experienced homeopath and begin treatment." To the next question, "Where can such be found in my area?" I have to reply with a pat answer. I live in the Saxon countryside and have little contact with colleagues from other regions, at least not so much that I can judge their competence. However, the address of various institutes that credentials homeopaths can be found via the internet.

I realize that I am walking a tightrope in linking homeopathic technicalities together with a discussion that has general appeal in one and the same book. One or the other discussion could prove either too superficial or too demanding. However, for myself the strategy makes sense on the whole. In addition it underscores my daily experience with patients, which is that some lay-persons are more knowledgeable concerning a subject that specially interests them than the doctors or naturopaths by whom they were advised in the course of treatment.

All that is needed for understanding is openness and a lack of bias. May all my readers possess these qualities today and for the rest of their lives.

Wildschütz, Autumn 2005
Peter Alex

Part 1: Theory & Practice

Infectious Disease

Counted among the principles of holistic theory and practice is the fact that phenomena must first be discriminated, if the meaning behind them is to be discerned. That the prevention of epidemics must include physical measures of hygiene is commonly known. From time immemorial epidemics only occur where very difficult social relations prevail; where there is hunger, privation and misery, most often accompanying or consequent to war. Thus the epidemic situation in Germany, as in Europe, eased considerably, owing simply to the subsequent improvement in living conditions. (Mistakenly, the leading producers of vaccines were held responsible for this decline, though this is supported neither by morbidity statistics nor by contemporary epidemic reports. Infectious diseases that have not been vaccinated against recede at the same rate or even quicker.)

Since bacteria and viruses are carriers of genetic information, and since this information is closely linked to the sickness of the infected person, a key can be found here to understand the phenomenon of an epidemic, or rather an infectious disease. Within a population there is always information circulating, which can make the susceptible person sick. As such, this is information with which we must to a greater or lesser extent concern ourselves.

In the tradition of Wilhelm Reich and Alexander Lowen, the German author and psychosomatic physician, Dr. Ruediger Dahlke, published several books on the topic of "the meaning of diseases and symptoms." For many common complaints Dr. Dahlke provided a lucid explanation as to what was to be learned on the mental plane from certain symptoms. Worth noting, however, is the fact that his books failed to provide any such explanation for collective problems, and thus for epidemics. Those explanations given in his reference work for scarlet fever or leprosy might occasionally accord with the individual level, but they don't account for the epidemic's appearance, and thus with the *collective* meaning of these infectious diseases.

We must, however, guard against the possibility that speculations on this level might turn into harmful stereotypes. In her seminal work

Disease as Metaphor, Susan Sontag points out that in the 19th century, "the notion that the disease fits the patients' character, as the punishment fits the sinner, was replaced by the notion that it expresses character." Noting that such notions are akin to blaming the victim, Sontag asserts that theories about the mental origin of disease are always an index of how much is <u>not</u> understood about its physical terrain. "Nothing," she writes, "is more punitive than to give a disease a meaning — that meaning being invariably a moralistic one." Any important disease whose causality is murky, and for which treatment is ineffectual, tends to be imbued with an excess of significance. For those who are concerned with the social aspect of Lyme disease, it would be useful to note the kinds of metaphors that currently clump around it. Within our own field of discourse we might begin with the Jungian homeopath Edward Whitmont, who speculated that Lyme disease arose from human-induced disturbances in the balance of Nature. As provocative as this insight may be, from there it is not such a big step to label individual sufferers as crass violators of the culture/nature boundary.

From these background considerations two questions come into focus:

- What role do bacteria play for life in general and for our human existence in particular?
- Why do the same bacteria cause grievous illness among some humans (and groups), while among others they have no effect at all?

Recommended reading for an understanding of evolution in general and also of our connection with bacteria is the recent book, *Microcosm*, by Lynn Margulis and Dorion Sagan. The authors note that, according to observed cell-counts, a human being consists of 91% bacteria cells and 9% animal cells.

Even this 9% of animal cells contains a multitude of organelles, which actually are bacteria like the mitochondria, that live within us on a symbiotic basis. Although it has been known since 1928 that these bacteria are essential for all animals as energy conduits, the molecular-genetic confirmation for this constitutes recent data. Mitochondria even have their own distinctive DNA, and they undergo division independent of host cell mitosis.

Bacterial cells 91%
Animal cells 9%

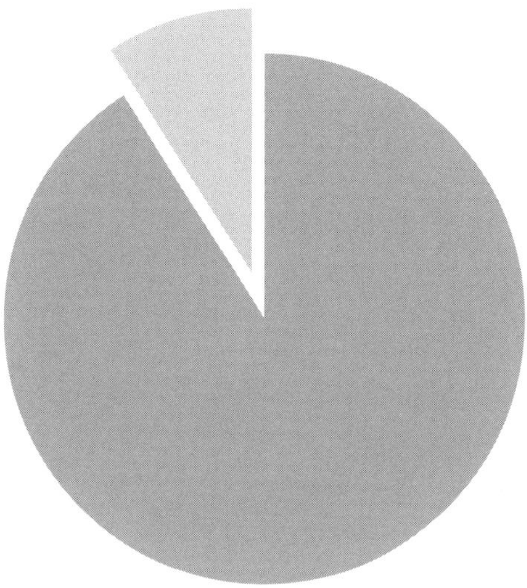

Much further developed is our symbiosis with previously flagellated bacteria capable of independent movement. These "bestowed" the microtubuli on us. The latter are small, motile organelles, which compose our ciliated epithelium. They are found for example in the bronchi and the fallopian tubes. They also provide locomotion for the sperm as bearers of the male hereditary code. The structure of these microtubuli has remained unchanged from the first bacteria that appeared more than two billion years ago down to the present time.

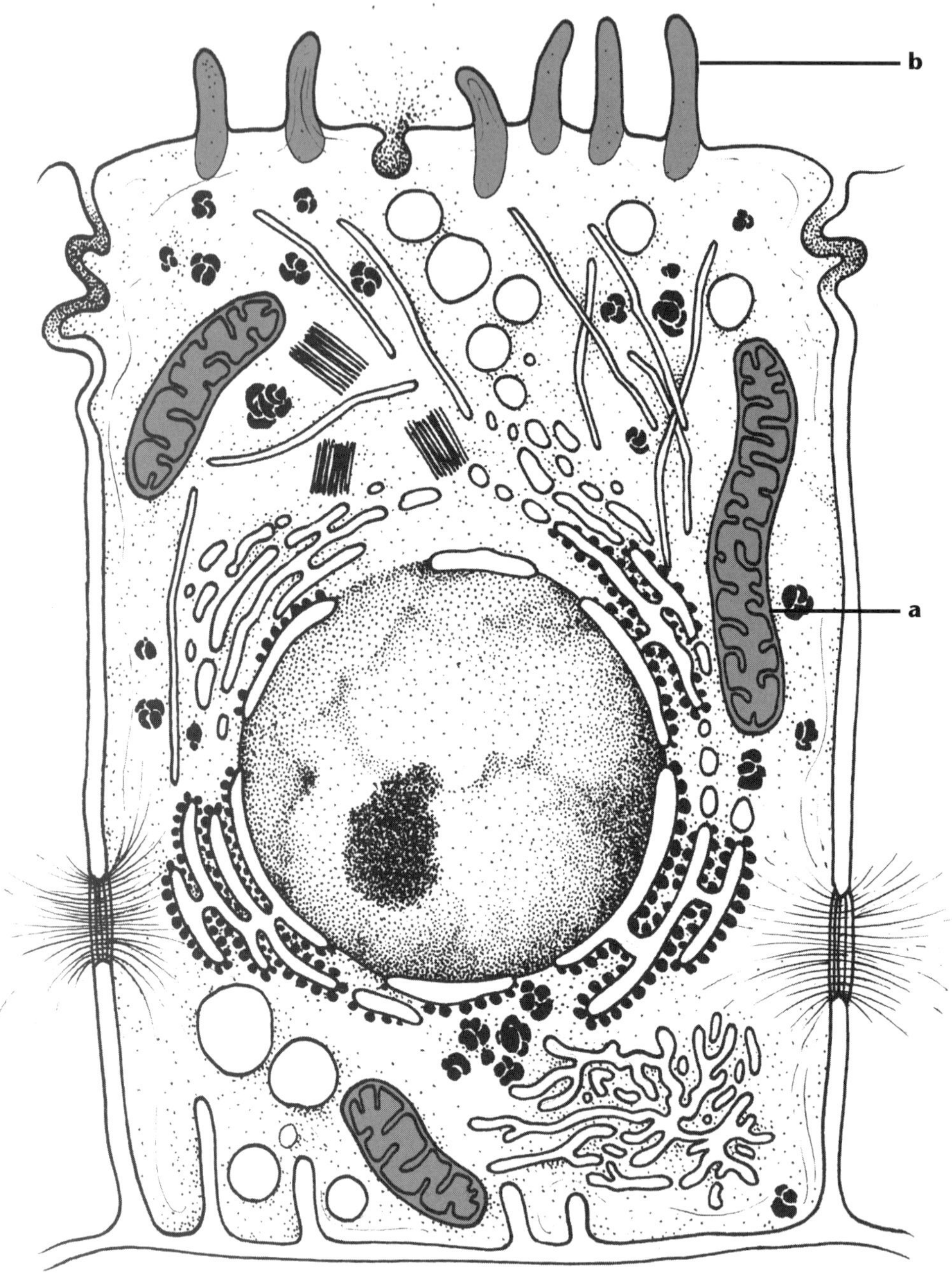

Schematic drawing of an animal (specifically human) cell. The mitochondria (a) and the microtubules (b) are parts of the cell where bacteria became symbiotically incorporated.

Conspicuously equipped with such flagellae are the contemporary bacteria of the aforementioned family of Spirochaetaceae, to which the genera *Borrelia* and *Treponema* belong. Just as much as the (phylogenetically later) mitochondria, it is recognized that close relatives of the Spirochetes have merged with us symbiotically, making important contributions to our evolution. While the mitochondria today can still be unambiguously identified as "guest bacteria," this is no longer possible in the case of the microbes, which in our mutual symbiosis conferred the microtubuli construct. Their DNA has in the meantime been completely incorporated into the human genome.

Molecular geneticists today maintain that it is improbable that phylogenesis can have fueled itself only through genetic exchange involved in the sexual reproduction of the higher organisms (where there is only a single such act per generation.) Bacteria, however, engage in genetic exchange on a continuous basis. Occurring as numerically superior symbiotes in all higher life forms, it is very probable that they have played a decisive role in the genetic diversity and thus the evolution of these organisms. Mitochondria and microtubuli are but two striking examples.

Incidentally, we should recall as accepted fact that it was the bacteria which bequeathed us the oxygen content of the atmosphere; and that it was also bacteria which ensured that its oxygen content didn't rise above 16%, beyond which most life forms could not survive. Bacteria made the soil on which our foodstuff thrives. Without bacteria there would be neither wine, nor beer, nor sauerkraut, let alone cheese and yoghurt. Bacteria are not only indispensable for the production of our daily bread, but also for its digestion. In addition, bacteria turn the products of our digestion into soil, rendering them available for life. In short, not only is life without bacteria unthinkable from a scientific perspective, for humanity it would become a veritable nightmare, if even for one moment we had to do without these tiny creators and sustainers.

Indeed, it is high time that we cease depicting bacteria as the enemy, something which has been encouraged by the pharmaceutical industry under the mentorship of Robert Koch and Louis Pasteur.

If we accept that all contemporary life-forms (ourselves included) represent a complex cellular bond of bacteria that have been increasingly integrated over billions of year, then there are two distinct conclusions to be drawn:

- we do not develop immunity to those bacterial populations which convey such critical information that we cannot afford to screen them out; and
- every single therapy directed against bacteria creates a disturbance; that is, it upsets the natural course of our existence.

Should we not respect the fact that we have evolved over 3.5 billion years by continuously incorporating genetically transmitted information which is predominantly bacterial in nature? If a principle has operated that long, it is not perhaps a basic law of life? And if that is so, what are the consequences for those who devote their lives to the observation and treatment of disease?

If it is in the nature of evolution to integrate information, this being evidently the basis for:

- development of higher forms; and
- adaptation to ever-changing environmental conditions,

then a therapy which is observant of life and which is keyed to the laws of life can only proceed in the same or a similar manner.

Certainly we proceed thus in the course of homeopathic treatment. We provide the organism with information which as much as possible resembles the disease itself, leaving no further role for the sickness-inducing code borne by the natural carrier. There is no further affinity between the organism and the disease. Of course, this applies just as well for epidemic diseases. Once the coding of the disease is known, then a homeopathic remedy — that is, a similar coding — can be successfully prescribed on a therapeutic basis to those already sick, or on a preventive basis to healthy persons threatened with infection. The bacteria disappear from the body, which is to say they cease colonizing it.

Over the 200-year history of homeopathic medicine, many remedies and prophylactics have been recognized as appropriate for certain epidemics. Every homeopath who practices according to the rules of their art can doubtless cite numerous such cases from their own clinical experience. Of these, the following list offers but a small selection.

Infectious Disease	Associated Bacterium	Homeopathic Remedies (Examples)
Scarlet fever	Streptococcus	Belladonna, Mercurius solubilis
Cholera	Vibrio cholerae	Camphora, Carbo vegetabilis, Cuprum
Tetanus	Clostridium tetani	Ledum palustre, Hypericum perforatum
Malaria	Plasmodium	Chininum sulphuricum
Whooping Cough	Bordetella pertussis	Drosera rotundifolia, Ipecacuanha
Diptheria	Coyrnebacterium diphtheriae	Phytolacca, Lac caninum
Lyme disease	Borrelia	Ledum palustre, Aurum arsenicosum

Classification and Cultural Symbolism of the Spirochetes

Resembling tightly coiled snakes, spirochetes are distinguished by certain unique structures in their cell walls, which are known as *axial filaments*. These consist of flagellae and are responsible for the organism's motility. Spirochetes can move agilely with great speed through viscous substances. Otherwise they are similar to other gram-negative bacteria. The cell bodies are formed from an elongated cylinder that is rolled up in a spiral fashion. Many spirochetes live as parasites in humans and animals. Others live independently in water or mud. All spirochetes are chemoheterotrophic; that is, they are dependent on organic substances for carbon take-up and energy production.

The species of *Leptospira* are distinguished from other members of the line by their requirement for oxygen in a gaseous form, which would kill most other species instantly.

Order: Spirochaetales
- *Family: Leptospiraceae*
  - *Genus: Leptospira*
    - *Species Leptospira interrogans* (Welch disease)
- *Family: Spirochaetaceae*
  - *Genus: Borrelia*
    - *Species: Borrelia burgdorferi* (Lyme disease)
  - *Genus: Treponema*
    - *Species: Treponema pallidum* (syphilis)
    - *Species: Treponema pertenue* (framboisia, or yaws)

Syphilis was known as "the great imitator" because its manifold symptomology mimicked other known diseases. Now Lyme disease occupies the same stage as 'the new imitator.' P.H. Durey observes: "When they first realized that Borreliosa was a disease which began on the skin and then progressed to the joints, they classified it as an imitator of other diseases, similar to the way they dealt with syphilis in an earlier time." And in this regard Sir William Osler noted that, "To comprehend syphilis, you have to master all of medicine."

Homeopathy recognizes *Mercury*, the chief remedy for syphilis, as the "great camouflage artist." Considering the close affinity between both species of spirochete, it shouldn't be surprising that the first Lyme disease patient, who turned up in France in 1922, demonstrated a weak positive on the syphilis test, and was thus — according to the procedure of that time — treated with arsenic compresses.

Many patients with Lyme disease are initially assigned other diagnoses, such as arthritis, juvenile arthritis, rheumatoid arthritis, fibromyalgia, chronic fatigue syndrome, multiple sclerosis, lupus erythematosus, first-stage ALS, Alzheimer's (also in its first stage), Crohn's disease, irritable bowel syndrome, as well as many other lesser known afflictions.

The symptomatic spectrum of Lyme disease is so confusing that one patient asserted: "A poorly informed doctor wrote in his book about Lyme disease that the more widely diversified and the more peculiar the symptoms, the more likely we are dealing with a psychosomatic problem; but I have to say, the more likely it is that we are dealing with Lyme disease." The issue has proven controversial. Some maintain that the disease is too frequently diagnosed, some that it is too seldom diagnosed, while others report frequent misdiagnoses.

About *Treponema pallidum*

- It was discovered in 1905 by the German zoologist, Fritz Schaudinn, who named it *Spirochaeta pallida*.
- The anaerobic *Treponema* species includes several spirochetes that can cause disease amongst humans. *Treponema pallidum* is the bacterium associated with syphilis, while *Treponema denticola*, *Treponema macrodentium* and *Treponema oralis* all exist in the human oral cavity in the transition zone between the teeth and the gums.
- As with the mycobacterial species that accompany tuberculosis, Treponemas have a very high lipid content, which is unusual for bacteria.
- *Treponema p.* accesses the body via skin lesions or the mucous membranes.
- It is easily killed with soap and water, with dryness, and by temperatures above 42° C.
- It cannot be grown in a cultured medium.

- Syphilis is diagnosed by means of serological procedures, dark-field microscopy, immunofluorescence testing, or by virtue of clinical findings.
- False-positive test results are caused: by other *Treponema* species; by smallpox vaccinations; by pregnancy; by cancer; by either acute or chronic infections such as mononucleosis or malaria; by certain long-term conditions (intravenous use of drugs, autoimmune diseases, cancer); and by old age.

the good news ...

The biblical figure of Job was probably the victim of a syphilitic infection. After losing both family and property, he became covered from head to foot with repulsive sores. At night the pains gnawed his bones, allowing him no rest. According to the Book of Job, the lesson he had to learn was that suffering in all its immediacy is a compelling and purifying experience for consciousness. It is not a punishment, despite the fact that Job pleaded his innocence and rebelled against the injustice of it all.

Carl Gustav Jung called syphilis "the poison of darkness." Nevertheless, there are some for whom darkness is an essential source of inspiration, as Deborah Hayden points out in her book, *The Pox: Genius, Madness, and the Secrets of Syphilis*. In Hayden's terms, it is through his search for creative powers that the syphilitic character makes a kind of Faustian pact[1], by which he endures pain and despair, so that he can experience periods of creative exuberance, enthusiasm, and joyful energy, the brilliance of which ushers in a new world-view. In certain cases it appears that syphilis can stimulate genius: "The heightened perception, the overwhelming insights, and the almost mystical knowledge that are experienced in these periods attain expression, so long as the precise medium of expression remains intact."

The French novelist, Guy de Maupassant (1850-1893), was beside himself with delight when he came down with syphilis in 1877. Joyfully he exclaimed: "I've got syphilis! At last! Not the contemptible clap, no, no, the Thing Itself, from which Francis I died. Syphilis, the Majestic ... and I am

[1] Faust, the chief character in Goethe's *Faust* and Thomas Mann's *Doctor Faustus*, presents an example of someone who is ready to trade his soul to the devil in exchange for creativity and boundless knowledge.

proud of it, goodbye and to hell with the bourgeoisie." It is very hard here to draw a dividing line between good and evil, because often it is equally difficult to separate madness and genius. Hayden maintains that the leap in the quality of Maupassant's literary production from the merely mediocre around 1876 to the heights of mastery in the short period after 1880 is evidence for an extraordinary activation of his brain cells.

Fyodor Dostoyevski (1821-1881) suffered from epilepsy and syphilis. Yet he wrote: "What does it matter that it has been called a disease? What difference does it make whether it is normal or abnormal, if upon reflection and in a healthy state I experience this moment as one of complete harmony and beauty? It provides me with experiences of vastness, richness and eternity, and reconciles me with everything, when this marvelous, sublime merger with the highest union in life overcomes me."

During the 1930s Hans Zinsser contended that the interaction of spirochetes and humans had made a significant contribution to the expressiveness of our species. If only we allow evolution to continue undisturbed, "at last a point would be reached, where the mutual accommodation would be so complete that the host would no longer show any signs of interference." If in future humanity can remain as "syphilized" as it was in the past, a condition could be reached a thousand years hence (as is already the case with mouse spirochetes), where for anyone in the fullness of life a peritoneal tap would reveal *Treponema pallidum*, to which the host would be altogether oblivious. To Zinsser's apparent regret, the prospects for the syphilization of humanity were ruined through treatment with arsenic preparations. "This could be a loss for civilization: it has often been argued that, since so many outstanding men have syphilis, some of the greatest human achievements in reality originated in brains that owe their ability to a stimulus in the early stage of a general deterioration." (Zinsser 1960)

... and the bad

Neurosyphilis was first clearly described at the beginning of the 19th century by physicians employed in the asylums of Paris. The "madness" was perceived to be on the increase soon after the Napoleonic wars, to the point where syphilis eventually became known as "the disease of the century." While the avant-garde regarded syphilis as a means to gain the drive and inexhaustible energy upon which genius thrives, for the great majority of the afflicted the disease was something to be kept secret. They converted sex into shame, pleasure into guilt, and a sorrowful life into an often-premature death. Firmly believing that syphilis originated in sin and depravity, the physicians of the time treated their neurosyphilitic patients as hopeless, immoral and brute paralytics.

Concealment is in the very nature of syphilis. After the initial chancres disappear, the disease goes into hiding in various parts of the body, either to re-emerge after decades of latency, or else to slumber for the remainder of the life of the person who has been infected.

In its emergence as much as its disappearance syphilis as a collective disease operates in a similar fashion. Medical historians recognize that syphilis first appeared during the invasion of Italy in 1494/95 by the army of Charles VIII of France. Within his army were Spanish soldiers, who had accompanied Columbus on his journey to the New World. It was these soldiers who brought syphilis back to Europe.

In referring to the "astonishing evolution of syphilis," Jared Diamond explains: "What we imply today by the word 'syphilis' are sores on the genitals and a very slowly developing disease, which after many years results in death for the untreated victims. However, according to the first descriptions of syphilis in Europe in 1495, vesicles would cover the body from head to toe, producing a situation where peoples' flesh actually peeled away from the bones, such that death ensued within a few months. By 1546 the disease had developed to the point where its symptoms are recognizable today. Evidently syphilis resembles myxomatosis, in that these particular spirochetes have evolved to the extent that they can permit their victims to stay alive longer, so that they can transmit their spirochete offspring to that many more victims."

It remains an open question, whether syphilis is actually a new character on the stage of human existence, or whether it existed back into antiquity. Ancient writings seem to support the latter view, as do recent discoveries in Africa. There they have found skeletal remains, dated 1.5 million years old, with markings on the arm and leg bones. The number and arrangement of these markings point to yaws as the cause. Similar bone markings have been found in south Italy on the thigh bones of *Homo erectus*, who is one-half million years old. This point to the reasonable conclusion that early humans, as they began spreading out over Africa, carried yaws with them, an infectious disease that is non-sexually transmitted.

Is it conceivable that syphilis evolved over a relatively short interval into a sexual disease? On this subject the biologist Christopher Wills writes: "We must begin to realize that in the case of syphilis we are dealing with the extreme of a continuum of disease symptoms, about which for the most part we know very little. They have plagued mankind and its related species for a very long time. Syphilis is simply the extreme manifestation of the attempt by a parasite to spread from one host to another."

We ourselves might note that this last viewpoint conveys the typical good/bad bias of reductionistic medicine. Very much prior to that, it would make sense to pose the question as to why syphilis did not harm the American aboriginals to the same degree. Why did they react to the spirochetes' codon in a way that was evidently quite different from the Europeans? Had they already so integrated this codon that they did not have to fall sick anymore? In their state of collective development did they no longer need that information? Or had its time simply not yet come?

What is Lyme Disease?

At the beginning of the 70's an unusual number of cases of juvenile rheumatoid arthritis were reported from the region around Old Lyme, Connecticut. From this town was derived the English name of the disease. Many of those affected said that they had noticed a skin outbreak before the joint pains set in, and a portion of these recalled tick bites in the past — in the very place where the skin lesions later made their appearance. In the beginning the disease manifested prominently in the late summer, during the period when ticks were normally at their maximum. Earlier reports of a skin disease that ran a similar course, called *acrodermatitis*, are available from the 19th century.

The bacterium infesting the ticks was named *Borrelia burgdorferi* after Dr. Willy Burgdorfer, the researcher who isolated the spirochete in 1981. This gave rise to its present name, *borreliosis*.[2] Subsequently cases began turning up all around the world with the exception of Australia. Even arctic birds carried the borrelia pathogen.

Borrelia burgdorferi, the genospecies found in the USA, is associated chiefly with the arthritic form of the disease, termed "Lyme arthritis." Prevalent at more northerly latitudes, *B. afzelli* is thought responsible for the progression into acrodermatis chronica atrophicans. *B. garinii*, the strain which appears in western Europe, is associated with a particularly severe neurological progression. However, the zones of contagion overlap.

Initially, the warmer regions of southern Germany were the more heavily infected, since ticks below a temperature of 10 C. are barely active, and most will freeze during the winter. Some biologists have claimed that the less severe winter weather of the past years is a cause for the explosive increase of *borrelia*-infected ticks.

In the meantime the contagion has since spread to all of Germany. This is verified by an official enumeration of recent infections state by state, which (without considering the considerable number of unreported or false negative cases) may lie around 250,000 instances per year. The region around Kraichgau in North Baden is most heavily affected, with

[2] Translator's note. In this text with rare exception *borreliosis* is rendered as *Lyme disease*, the former disease-term being unfamiliar to English-speaking readers.

Hassler et al. finding fully 17% of the population infected. Regarding the official count, a statistical artifact arises in the fact that after the initial skin manifestations, the condition often continues untreated on a subclinical basis, only to break out under immunodeficient conditions months or years later with aggravated symptomatology.

In her monograph on the subject, Fust warned in strong terms about the possibility of tick bites in the winter months. That is the season when people gather Christmas boughs in which living ticks may have taken up residence. The general reaction to this and similar warnings was one of denial. Indeed, the epidemiological concern with Lyme disease suffered a setback, such that in the majority of German states there was no official obligation to report the disease until mid-2002. Anyone who came down with an exotic infectious disease, after (say) a ten-year sojourn in the tropics, was obliged to report to the health authorities, but not so for those who had fallen prey to the epidemic Lyme phenomenon.

People shouldn't count on their physician or naturopath to know more about Lyme disease than they do themselves. Even today, twenty years after the identification of the *Borrelia* spirochete and more than thirty years after the first modern description of the disease, it often happens that patients may consult a doctor who is completely uninformed about the disease. Unfortunately, such encounters still occur with some frequency.

For those who have been recently bitten, blood tests are taken to identify antibodies, while at the same time antibiotic therapy is initiated. After two weeks a further antibody test is made and — this proving negative — another success for antibiotics is announced. Of course this is pure humbug. Even in lay magazines it is plain to read that antibodies appear at the earliest four weeks and even later following a tick-bite. This means that any money spent either for the test or for the antibiotic treatment (let alone the damage to health) is simply thrown out the window.

During the summer of 2001, at a clinic specialized in neurology it could still happen that a sick person with clear indications of neuroborreliosis (see Case 10) could spend six weeks there, undergoing every conceivable (and expensive!) examination, without anyone thinking to perform a comparatively simple test for Lyme antibodies.

Since the Lyme spirochete (as with many other infectious diseases) confers no immunity after a bout with the disease, a person can be newly infected with the microbe on each further exposure.

The transmission route of the infected tick leads from small rodents or ungulates (hence the American name, *deer tick*), through grass-stalks and bushes, etc., to which the ticks adhere. It finally reaches humans either directly or via the rambling of a dog or other domesticate. To be sure, among humans exposed skin surfaces make access easier for the ticks (see also the discussion of *Prevention*), but they also succeed amongst thickly haired animals, where they can find, as in the teat area, a place to make a puncture.

The notion, previously widespread, that ticks drop from above onto their victims, has now been discarded. In no field study have ticks been found higher than one meter above the ground. In their most active mode the creatures crawl from below to above. Ticks prefer thin, hairless places on the skin, which are hard to reach by affected humans or animals. When a suitable animal presents itself to the parasite, they are led via chemical and thermic pathways to these sites.

In Germany as well as North America people ordinarily speak of "tick bites." More accurately the tick actually *stings* its victim. Ticks have no teeth, but rather pierce the skin like a mosquito. While sucking blood the tick buries its sucking apparatus so firmly in the skin that any careless pulling or scratching will more likely tear off the body, while leaving the head behind (in this connection see also *Prevention Using Homeopathy* below.) As with most blood-sucking parasites, ticks inject an anti-coagulant enzyme into the puncture site, allowing them to suck for an extended period (if undisturbed, the tick's feast can last for 1-2 days.)

Laboratory research in the USA has established that it takes 48 hours at the earliest for the borrelia bacteria to transfer from the tick to the host organism. In my experience none of those affected observed such a long period of infestation. More than one-third of the patients seen in my practice are quite sure that they were never bitten by a tick at all. On account of these conflicting claims, I am of the opinion that among humans the time-span from the tick bite to the transference of bacteria is either shorter than in the laboratory, or else there are pathways of transmission other than by tick puncture. The latter conjecture gains support from observations that a Lyme-type erythema migrans can appear at the site of a mosquito bite (Melhorn 2000). Other observers contend that the tiny millimeter-long tick larvae, whose bite is rarely noticed, could be the cause for infections that are not apparently due to ticks.

Since mosquitoes in our latitudes are also known to carry other epidemic diseases (for example, myxomatosis amongst rabbits), the suspicion arises that they also have their part to play in spreading Lyme disease. It is to be hoped that this might be researched from the epidemiological side. (Of course, to look for Lyme disease in a swarm of mosquitoes would not be a labour of love!)

Yet to be researched is the role of cat fleas as a disease vector.

For the time being we may assume on a conjectural basis that Lyme disease has something to do with our modern lifestyle, with some sort of imbalance in our social, emotional, physical, or mental hygiene, which makes it so easy in turn for these minuscule beings to attach themselves to us and then infest our system. Every disease, every epidemic has its correspondences on other planes, which is, so to speak, a collective message or signal to the affected group that something is not right. What that might be exactly requires further research, conducted – as Susan Sontag would urge — in a spirit of compassion rather than censure. I invite interested colleagues to work together to that end. An essential step towards understanding this phenomenon could be to prove the *Borreliosis nosode* as well as the chief vector, the *Ixodes rizinus* tick, in homeopathic potency.

Further, we have the interesting observation by Edward Whitmont, that — at least in the USA until the mid-90s — the Lyme zone is to be found encircling the conurbations. Urban as well as industrial centres, together with extensive unsettled regions, show no evidence of Lyme infestation. On this matter Whitmont's theory was that humans in their striving to live in nature — without, however, actually allying with her (reckless suburbanization has caused immense damage to the biotopes that had previously been unaffected) — unleashed this disturbance in the balance of nature. Unfortunately our colleague died before he had the opportunity to substantiate his theory.

The accelerating destruction through heedless sprawl (paving-over of open spaces, channeling or diverting rivers, clear-cutting of forests, destruction of animal habitats) left a surviving biotope that served as a sensitive indicator — and one that swung in our disfavour. Not by chance does the initial expression of Lyme disease take the form of circular skin outbreaks! *As above so below:* the fundamental hermetic law cannot be more clearly expressed. As it goes with nature as a whole, so it goes with each and every one of us. We mustn't forget that those of us who want to go live in the woods, who want to live on the outskirts of the city or beyond, do so because they love nature. They want to hear frogs croaking and bluebirds singing, and to watch how the fox and the hare say goodnight. But they also want to roll smoothly into the garage with the second car, answer their mobile phone on the terrace, and have a supermarket nearby, where a mango costs less than a dollar. All of this is obviously too much for our environment. That *too-muchness* we know in homeopathic terms as *sycosis*. Many Lyme patients manifest sycotic symptoms, as the case descriptions in Part 3 will make clear. Possibly in this way we draw closer to the root of all evil than we would like.

The natural balance threatens to tip, analogous to one of the head symptoms of Lyme disease in its neurological form. There one finds a tremendous reeling vertigo, such as appears in only a few other diseases.

Synergistic Factors in the Origin of Lyme Disease

Several instances of Lyme disease, which resisted a successful resolution for some time, provided significant insights that I would like to bring to the attention of the reader, in order to establish whether other patients or therapists have had similar experiences.

In four neurological cases of Lyme disease I have ascertained that the affected person, right at the point when the pains began, used a mobile phone employing pulsed high-frequency transmissions. Either that, or directly in or near their home a transmitter such as this had been put into service. The patients found themselves in neurological treatment for months or years with no benefit. In no case was neuro-borreliosis diagnosed, before I initiated the research, so that it cannot be said what came first: the electromagnetic field pollution, or the Lyme infection. In those cases where the patients installed a telephone with above-ground equipment, the homeopathic treatment brought about a sudden improvement (see Case 12.)

We are afforded an astonishing parallel here between, on the one hand, the typical close-meshed web of the mobile phone network creating neuro-pathogenic wave-patterns in our environment; and, on the other, the demonstrated efficacy of homeopathically-prepared spider poisons among Lyme patients. Pointing in the same direction is the fact that the chief vector of *Ixodes rizinus* happens to be a spider.

Several cases point to a link between Lyme disease and vaccination. An American microbiologist has recently isolated a botulin-like toxin as a metabolic product of the borrelia bacterium. Botulin toxin is better known as the metabolic product of *Clostridium botulinum,* a spore-forming bacterium; it is moreover the strongest bacterial poison known to man. Another bacterium of the same genus, *Clostridium tetani*, plays an accompanying (not causative) role in tetanus. As we know, tetanus vaccine, which is administered with increasing frequency by allopathic medicine, is involved as a causal agent in the origin of chronic neurological diseases. The connection with multiple sclerosis has been frequently demonstrated. In a case from my own practice a young woman became ill with multiple sclerosis shortly after receiving a second tetanus shot. As we know, many neurological cases of Lyme disease are misdiagnosed by specialists as multiple sclerosis. It would thus be desirable to establish which of these factors exerts an influence. But here we need more accurate observations using a consistent recording format.

Clinical Expressions of Lyme Disease

The clinical expressions of Lyme disease are numerous and often non-specific. If the infection is to develop into a full-blown case, as with all infectious diseases there must first be some weakened power of resistance in the susceptible host organism. In the final analysis it makes no sense to pose the question, *Which came first, the disease or the bacterium?* since we are concerned here with a synchronous and not a causal relationship.

As with syphilis (at least as it pertains to the associated germ), allopathic clinicians distinguish three stages:

1. The localized stage with a fairly typical skin outbreak, known as erythema migrans. Most patients who have suffered a tick bite, recall a more or less large red ring around the tick's entry-point. At the same time there can appear non-specific infections, such as fever, flu-like symptoms, fatigue, and swelling of the lymph nodes in the region of the puncture.
2. For weeks or months the infection may remain unnoticed, or else the person affected makes no connection with their current illness, because the symptoms are non-specific. Sometimes for the first months or years after the infection, there is no discernible symptomatology. But as the disease continues to burrow in, eventually it takes the form of a chronic arthritis affecting every possible joint, sometimes with and sometimes without identifiable rheumatoid blood factors.
3. In the third stage the disease centers on the nervous system, manifesting as a nervous attack (often recognized as neuralgic pains, paralysis, or vertigo), or as acrodermatitis chronica atrophicans.

Recently bacteriologists have considered further serotypes as the pathogen responsible for these various syndromes. However, from the viewpoint of holistic medicine it doesn't make much sense to adopt this classification. One can possibly provide opinions concerning the anticipated length of treatment, but even here there is no sure way of knowing in a substantial number of cases.

In my practical experience cases in clinical stage 2, the arthritic, return to health more quickly than those in stage 3, the neurological. This is something upon which Hering's Rule sheds some light, for the nervous system viewed as a whole represents a deeper level of the being than the articular system.

On the miasmatic level we regard joint diseases, to the extent that they are deforming, as more sycotic than syphilitic. During the degenerative neurological phase the syphilitic nature comes to the fore, with unfortunately a reduced possibility of healing.

Proving of value in my practice has been Friedrich Graf's clinical classification of Lyme disease into its *dermal*, *articular* and *neurological* forms. With Lyme disease, a clinical differential diagnosis is important, as much for the prognosis as for the course of therapy, in case some aetiological factor other than a tick bite may be involved.

Dermal

- erythema, resembling herpes infections.
- allergic skin reactions through contact with plant parts, animal hair, insect bites or chemical substances
- infestation with other parasites (especially during visits to the tropics)

Articular

- hereditary tendency to rheumatic joint diseases, especially after the patient or their predecessors suffered gonorrheal or chlamydial infections (sycotic arthritis)
- acquired rheumatic symptoms following insults to the immune system (for example, vaccinations)

Neurological

- multiple sclerosis (often as a delayed consequence of an auto-immune disease, for example, following vaccinations, particularly for tetanus)
- meningitis and encephalitis arising from other infectious diseases
- other neurological syndromes, for example Menière's disease
- facial neuralgia: previous inflammations, dental treatments, pernicious dental fillings, nervous inflammations in other contexts

- neurological disturbances from mobile phone radiation (increasingly experienced in my practice)

As yet there is no homeopathic remedy picture for Lyme disease, but in the meantime the extensive case-literature can offer a provisional construct.

What we have done below is to organize the reported symptomatology according to the standard framework of a homeopathic Materia Medica, beginning with the mind and proceeding downwards through the organ systems to the extremities.

MIND

General Picture

In one U.S. study of 27 patients with advanced neuroborreliosis, 33% were depressed, based on their scores on the Minnesota Multiphasic Personality Inventory. The majority (89%) of these 27 patients also had evidence of a mild encephalopathy, characterized by memory loss (81%), excessive daytime sleepiness (30%), extreme irritability (26%), and word finding difficulties (19%). Controlled studies indicate significantly more depression among patients with late Lyme disease than among healthy controls or other chronically ill patients.

A diagnostic indicator pointing to Lyme disease as the cause of the depression and irritability might be concomitant memory loss, word finding problems, or a concomitant neuropathy.

Hypersensitivity

Light

- Photophobia [keynote]; must wear sunglasses or snow goggles, even indoors and at night.
- Feeling of faintness or dizziness from exposure to fluorescent lights, making it difficult to go to supermarkets or other public places.
- Panic attacks triggered by light stimulation, esp. flickering bright lights.
- Nausea from flickering bright lights (fluorescent lights, TV or computer screens, strobe lights during EEG testing, or the headlights of cars moving in the opposite line of traffic.)

Sound

- Ordinary conversation perceived as deafening; wears head–phones and puts pillows over his head to block out the sound. To one woman even the sound of another person's breathing seemed unbearably loud. In her case, the sound sensitivity also included vertigo, nausea and nystagmus in response to sounds. Any sudden sound, like the phone ringing, and certain household sounds, like the running to tap water, could cause her to fall or retch. This peculiar short-circuiting of the inner ear's auditory and vestibular functions is known as the Tullio phenomenon. This phenomenon has been deemed pathognomic for syphilis but, as it appears, can occur in Lyme disease as well. It thus provides one more example of the 'new great imitator,' Lyme disease, imitating the old 'great imitator,' syphilis.

Odor

- Smells seem overly intense and noxious.

Taste

- Foods taste abnormally sour or bitter
- Or the reverse: loss of taste *on the left side of tongue.*

Touch

- Regional or generalised hyperaesthesia of skin to touch or temperature.
- Sensitivity to touch: "The bed sheet resting lightly on my toe would make the toe ache, like a toothache." "Even the thinness of a sheet was too painful for my legs."

Vibration

- Abnormally heightened vibratory sense; e.g. thinks car were vibrating with unusual violence.

Emotional Lability / Mood Swings / Irritability

- Accompanied by headache and stiff neck.
- Sudden, intense irritability from sensory stimulation (sound, touch, light) or occurring unprovoked and inexplicably.

- Sudden, unprecedented fits of violence.
- Uncontrollable outbursts: "A women, typically reserved and eager to please, became uncontrollably irritable one day at work and found herself yelling at her boss in a most uncharacteristic fashion."
- Suddenly bursting into tears over trifles.
- Fluctuations from marked agitation to severe depression with suicidal threats.
- Rapid mood swings, from grandiosity to sudden tearfulness.
- Violence: striking children and breaking furniture.

Homicidal ideation and compulsive behavior occur in some of these patients. Some adult patients describe struggling to not act on these urges. **When patients act on a homicidal urge; more commonly, a child who attacks a sibling.** Dissociative episodes sometimes occur with these patients, occasionally accompanied by aggressive behavior and memory loss.

Cognitive Impairment — Lyme Fog

- Brain fag; problems with facial recognition.
- Spaced out, as if in a fog.
- Difficulty remembering details such as names or appointment times. Engaged in new compensatory behavior, such as daily list making.
- Compensatory compulsions are common in an effort to compensate for the memory deficits. [Lyme disease] patients generally come to the office disorganized [despite a supreme effort to be organized], unable to give a coherent history. They will bring copious notes, which are invariable in the wrong order. As one patient expressed it, "I used to have a quick mind and a good memory. Now I am dependent on notes plastered everywhere so I can remember things."
- Short-term memory problems, word-finding difficulties, dyslexia, problems with calculations or inability to concentrate. Many Lyme patients state, "I feel like I have become dyslexic." Impairment of reading comprehension is an earlier sign with the later addition of auditory comprehension difficulties. Acquired left/right confusion is seen with some of these patients displaying what appears to be

> an acquired Gerstmann's syndrome [Gerstmann's syndrome: the inability to perceive a stimulus applied to the fingers, impairment of the ability to write, inability to do simple mathematical problems, and confusion of laterality of body] or some variant of this syndrome. They have problems with calculations and often complain of errors when trying to calculate their checkbooks. Fluency of speech is a very significant problem. When interviewing these patients, this is a clearly evident symptom. Stuttering is seen in many of these patients.

A boy, five years of age, said, "I would mix up stories and get cranky. I tried to tell Mom that my brain was 'sticky', but she didn't know what I meant. It didn't hurt, it just wouldn't work. I would climb up on the sink and put a wet washcloth on my head. In those days my behaviour was hyperactive and I would stutter."

Another patient says, "The kicker, though, was the virtually inexplicable difficulty in writing, typing, speaking, and thinking. I'd use the wrong letters, hit the wrong keys, stutter, reverse things, and find myself unable to say the right word. Everyone does this occasionally, but this was consistent and unrelenting. I felt like something poisonous had taken over my brain."

In interviews, patients with Lyme encephalopathy tend to be vague and disorganized in narrating the history of their illness. This is despite their close attention to their symptoms and having recounted them many times before. Although in most cases memory of discreet events — tests, dates, diagnoses, responses to medications — is intact, the patient is unable to recall them spontaneously or organize them in temporal order. They may be unclear as to their chief complaint. They may completely lose track of what they were saying, sometimes repeatedly, or of what the question was. They may get off on a tangent and have trouble re-orienting themselves. Frequent prompting and refocusing will be necessary. Beginning the interview with an open-ended question like "Tell me what the problem is" will allow these qualities to become clear.

However, their experience is different from that of ADD, in that rather than having the experience that there are many thoughts competing for attention, the Lyme patient has difficulty bringing *any* thought into clear focus. They experience difficulty thinking. One patient described it as the universe ending six inches from his face. He couldn't process information that was not immediately apparent, immediately experienced. Another said that when he tries to think about something, or figure something out, all he can do is repeat the question — he can't get to the meaning. One patient, a physician, described it as a *mental intention tremor — the more she tries to focus on something the more out of focus it becomes.*

Mistakes in speaking and/or writing

- "Patients with no prior history of dyslexia have found themselves writing letters backwards, reversing numbers or routinely reversing the first and second letters of a word."
- Mistakes in time: says "tomorrow" instead of "yesterday" and vice versa.

Spatial and positional disorientation ("spatial dyslexia")

- Loses his way in well-known streets. "I was getting lost in my neighborhood when I tried to drive." "I was getting lost driving to places that I had been to hundreds of times." "I forgot when I was on my way home."
- Difficulty with spatial awareness of where front and back doors are in one's own house.
- Disturbed sense of position. "Repeatedly bumps into things on the left side of her body, drops things from her left hand despite having no weakness in that hand, and occasionally places objects several inches short of a table edge with the result that they fall to the floor.
- Disturbed sense of position, esp. in hands; grasps the air when reaching for objects.
- Spatio-temporal distortions: "Everything around me looked strange. The people sounded like cackling geese. Everyone looked like they were in fast motion, like someone had sped up the projector. Every time I turned, I was dizzy and disoriented. I was sweating and completely lost."

Hallucinations

- Musical hallucinations with a sudden onset, taking the form of patriotic or operatic music.

- "I had both visual and auditory hallucinations. I heard phones ring when there were none. I saw shadows twist into menacing shapes. I heard voices talking. At night, I saw flashing lights fill my vision, and my ears were constantly buzzing with static and ringing. I felt for the first time that I might be truly going mad."
- Upon waking at night: "A skeleton hallucination in black and white, looking at me, grinning a very toothy smile, head cocked, propped up by one arm."

Intrusive thoughts and images

- Intrusive obsessional thoughts with efforts to stem such; horrific images of killing others; excessive bathing.
- Intrusive images that are generally aggressive but sometimes can be sexual or otherwise. Occasionally these images are of a homicidal nature.
- Chaotic processing: "My mind was a hopeless jumble of uncontrolled thoughts — images and sounds that haunted me. It was as if several minds had been merged into one, and there was no way to sort the images."

Fears

- Chronic morbid dread of vomiting (without actual emesis.)
- Panic attacks in sleep: "I woke up several times in pain and experiencing panic attacks."

CHILDREN

"The majority, over ninety percent, of the children that we have treated complain of headache. The headache, in a few cases, has been very acute accompanied by papilloedema [oedema of the optic disk] but in the majority of cases the headache comes on gradually, becomes quite persistent and does not respond to over-the-counter analgesics. In addition to the headache, the children complain of photophobia, dizziness, a stiff neck, backache, somnolence and, those that are in school have problems with memory and difficulty concentrating. Some patients have developed progressive weakness. The parents complain that pre-schoolers develop mood swings and become very irritable and they see a personality change. Among the children that are school age and those who are in adolescence, chest pain is a very frequent complaint. At least seventy percent have complained of chest pain. About fifty percent have complained of abdominal pain. More than half the children have arthralgia usually involving the knee and sometimes the wrist. Other complaints include palpitations, tingling, numbness, rashes that come and go, usually malar [cheek] rashes, and sore throats that are excruciatingly painful.

"It is easy to see how this long list can be very non-specific, such that many of these children are thought to have functional problems."

GENERALS

Typical Combination of Features

- Joint pain + major cognitive dysfunction (esp. short-range memory) + major sleep disturbances + terrible fatigue + sensory hyperacuity.

Alternating States

- Perplexing fluctuation in symptoms. Spry and energetic one day, drained and confused the next. May be brought on by exertion, stress, or exposure to sensory stimuli, or come without apparent cause. Cannot make plans due to the unpredictable nature of the fluctuations. "I thought I was slowly going crazy, never knowing what the next day would bring."
- Days of near-normality alternate with days of profound debility. "Days of hope and black despair coupled together."
- The symptoms shift in kaleidoscopic fashion from one hour to the next in the same patient and seldom present identically in two different individuals.

Suddenness

- All of a sudden suicidal.
- Sudden worsening of symptoms.
- Sudden inability to remember how to transfer calls [in a woman who had been a telephone switchboard operator for 20 years.]

- Worse by any sudden sound.
- Sudden intense irritability.
- Sudden soreness of sinuses and throat, at times disappearing, only to become sore again in a seemingly rhythmic way.
- Sudden, complete inability to swallow.
- Awakened in the middle of the night by severe arthritic pains over entire body. Pain sudden, dramatic, and excruciating. Pain gone when waking the next morning.
- Sudden changes in stool consistency, from normal to putty-like to constipation, where stools have to be removed mechanically, etc.
- Sudden arrhythmia.
- Sudden falling to the ground.
- Sudden paralysis. "As I stood in front of the bathroom sink brushing my teeth, I suddenly lost the use of my right arm and hand. A quivery, ticklish feeling traveled like lightning from the shoulder to the fingertips; paralyzed, the arm dropped down into the sink, hit the enamel hard and broke the skin.

Neurological

- Left-sided hemiparesis when waking up. "The left side of my face was paralyzed with the numbness extending to the left side of my tongue and down my throat. Also, my left side felt weaker and my left lung felt somehow affected — cold and heavy."
- Intermittent paraesthesias.
- Nerve pains severe, *burning*, tearing, migrating, with characteristic exacerbation at night.
- Clumsiness. Ataxia is common in these patients who are often clumsy, which leads to frequent accidents.
- The close resemblance between neuroborreliosis and certain neurological conditions has been explained thus: "When the human brain becomes inflamed, cells called macrophages respond by releasing a neurotoxin called quinolinic acid. This toxin is also elevated in Parkinson's Disease, MS, ALS, and is responsible for the

dementia that occurs in AIDS patients. What quinolinic acid does is stimulate neurons to repeatedly depolarize. This eventually causes the neurons to demyelinate and die." People with elevated quinolinic acid have short-term memory problems.

Energy

- Debilitating fatigue. "Too fatigued and sore to even think about moving around."
- Debilitating fatigue with periodic attacks of left-sided paralysis. The best description I can think of for the misery of acute Lyme disease is a combination of debilitating mononucleosis and severe arthritis in the knees and elbows.

Sleep — Night Aggravation

- Excessive daytime sleepiness. "Cannot sleep at night, cannot wake up during the day."
- Falling asleep while talking with others.
- Falling asleep at work.
- Narcolepsy. "At first, I would fall asleep spontaneously and unpredictably a few times a week, but over the next three months it climbed to four hundred times a day. I would fall when this happened."
- Apnoea: a sudden 'gasping' for air just before falling asleep.
- Sleeping disorder. A 13-year old boy "would thrash around at night disrupting his bedding, knocking over lamps and rearranging things during the night. I never actually saw any of these episodes but saw the result of them in the morning." "When I did sleep, it was a tortured sleep where I would toss and turn and tear at my covers. I despised warmth and craved cold. My bed in the morning would look like a war zone." "In the beginning, I was horrified to awaken knowing that I was still alive and had not died in my sleep. What a great cop-out, I would think, except the nightmares were actually worse than reality." "Woke up angry in the night that I hadn't just died."
- Night terrors. "I experienced night terrors, where friends that had died in the last twenty years gathered around my bed nightly,

smiling and waving for me to come with them ... I hated to go to sleep at night because of my dead friends appearing."

- Early morning insomnia with nightmares.
- Sleeplessness due to pain in kidneys.
- Sleeplessness from stabbing pain in feet.

Pains

- Burning [pain] is quite specific [to neuroborreliosis]; the patient describes a sensation that a blowtorch is burning the skin.
- Feeling as if muscles and nervous system were on fire. "The burning pain in my spine was so bad that I broke out in sweats day and night."
- Sharp shooting or stabbing pains.

Food and Drink

- Anorexia.
- Eating disorders are common. Invariably these patients either gain or lose weight. Sometimes massive weight gain is also seen.
- Increased thirst.
- Intolerance for alcohol. Most patients state, "I don't drink anymore."
- Exaggerated symptoms or heavy hangover from alcohol.

Temperature

- Great chilliness.
- Low body temperature [slightly below normal].
- Profuse sweating.
- Unexplained sweats. Night sweats. Sweating even in cool temperatures.

Weather

- Symptoms < in low pressure weather systems.

Miscellaneous

- Lymphocytoma [small solitary bluish-red plaque or nodule], particularly at ear lobes or nipples.
- Delayed development; failure to thrive in infants.

LOCALS

Vertigo

- Sensation of whirling motion, either of oneself or of external objects.
- Menière's disease.
- Vertigo with drop attacks of the Tumarkin type. [During Tumarkin's episodes or Tumarkin's otolithic crisis, patients suddenly fall to the ground without prior warning and without losing consciousness. Thought to be caused by a sudden change of the otolithic mass, the condition is not uncommon in the later stages of Menière's disease.]
- Motion sickness.
- Balance severely off; would fall when closing eyes.
- Vertigo from even slightly turning head: "The world would swim if I just moved my eyeballs."
- Floor feels as if it were rolling beneath the feet, or as if one were on an elevator or a boat, going up and down in the waves.

Head

- Headache, frontal or occipital, of intermittent duration and fluctuating intensity.
- Feeling of pressure behind eyes, pain < moving eyes.
- Sore/tender areas on skull/scalp area.
- Pressure migrating from vertex to occiput when turning head. "When I would move my head, there was a disturbing gurgle as if I heard bubbles move around inside my head."

Eyes and Vision

- Conjunctivitis
- Intermittent diplopia and visual blurring.
- Diplopia and vertigo and nystagmus.
- Triplopia in right eye.
- Sparks, spots, waves, floaters before eyes.
- Sensation of a foreign body in eye(s) [keratitis]
- Twitching.

- Bloodshot eyes.
- Vision reduced to a circle directly in front of eyes; peripheral vision just a blurry swirling mess of lights and images.
- Afterimage. "Seeing 'trails' of objects, e.g. my own moving limbs or doorways I walked through."

Hearing

- Impaired hearing (bilateral) and fatigue, headache, or arthritis.
- Hearing loss and tinnitus.

Face

- Bilateral facial nerve palsy.
- Muscle twitches in face.
- Pain in face, teeth, articulation of jaw, and masticator muscle.
- Swelling around eyes.
- Facial redness.
- Facial paraesthesias: "My chin hurt and felt 'ticklish' — as if something were blowing on it."
- Audible clicking of jaw when speaking or eating.
- Itching: "Around my mouth, all around the lips and down into the chin, a vibrating, biting, humming itch, as though there were a thousand bees swarming over my lips and the majority of them were stinging."

Mouth

- Numbness/tingling of face or tongue.
- Weakness of the tongue.
- Sore spots on tongue.
- Speech: slow and labored; slurred; poorly articulated.

Throat

- Must drink in order to swallow food.

Urogenital

- Irritable bladder; trouble starting/stopping; frequent urination; voiding dysfunction.
- Urinary retention followed by paralysis of lower limbs.
- Numbness of genitals.

Chest

- Short stabbing pains in chest lasting only seconds.
- Dry, non-productive cough.
- Awakening in middle of night with chest pains and pain and tingling down the left arm
- Sensation as if hot water were being poured into lungs.

Back

- Stiffness of nape of neck, with headache, pain in joints and/or muscles, or fatigue.
- Weakness in nape of neck.
- Tired feeling between shoulder blades, as if neck wouldn't support weight of head.
- Jabbing pain in the back as if being kicked in the kidneys.

Extremities

- Wandering joint/muscle pains without swelling, lasting hours or days in a given location.
- Pain in joints, only on motion.
- Joints sensitive to pressure.
- Localised joint pains/swelling involving mostly the knee(s), and to a far lesser extent the ankles, shoulders, and elbows.
- Paraesthesias: "I kept looking down at my upper arms to brush off the hair or cobwebs on them, and realized there was nothing there."
- Sensation as of a band pulled tightly around right lower arm halfway between wrist and elbow.

- Tendon problems: hands/fingers temporarily lock into unusual positions.
- Carpal tunnel syndrome and numbness of fingers, < during sleep or using hands.
- Intention tremor hands.
- Fingers on both hands fumble and cannot pick up small objects.
- White spots on fingernails; ridges; brittle nails.
- Deep, aching, burning pains in the hamstring muscles when sitting; sits on the very edge of a seat; cannot bear touch or slightest pressure on hamstrings.
- Leg joints give out, or wobble, rubbery legs. Unable to walk.
- Sensation of a tourniquet wrapped around right leg.
- Restless legs at night in bed, resulting in sleeplessness.
- Throbbing pain in ankles and in long bones in calves and shins. "Not an ache, but a feeling that someone had scraped the skin away, thrown salt into the raw tissue, then set it on fire."
- Severe pain in balls of feet; painful to put any weight on feet.

Skin

- Warm, wet, or cold sensations on skin.
- Regional or generalized hyperaesthesia of skin to touch or temperature.
- Excessively itchy skin. Urticaria.

Allopathic Prevention and Treatment

The pharmaceutical industry has been promising for years that it was right on the verge of a breakthrough in the search for a vaccine that would confer immunity against Lyme disease. Though happily not permitted in Germany, in America early generations of Lyme vaccines elicited the very syndrome that they were meant to protect against, and were duly taken off the market. This was no surprise for those familiar with immunology and vaccine iatrogenesis, since with all crude inoculations one must be prepared for the so-called *Pitcairn effect*. Vaccinations, which prevent the appearance of an acute form of infectious disease, lead regularly to the development of a chronic form of the corresponding disease amongst those who have been vaccinated. Since the chronic disease often has no obvious link to the acute disease — nothing that the vaccinated person can point to — it is given another name and thus the connection with the vaccination is further obscured.

The treatment for Lyme disease using antibiotics is just as double-edged. While in the short term it reduces *borrelia* in the blood count, in the long term it ravages the immune system. A preventive round of antibiotics may leave those who have become infected symptom-free, yet in all probability they would suffer nothing or only the relatively mild skin form anyway. Nothing at all is proved in either case, since with every infection the development of disease symptoms depends ultimately on the strength of the individual's immune system.

In my homeopathic practice, dealing with the damage which antibiotic treatment causes the immune system sometimes proves just as difficult as treating the original symptoms following the tick bite.

An established infection often cannot be eradicated with antibiotics. In the case of Lyme disease, shortly after the bite (a few hours to two days), it can be demonstrated that once lodged within the cell, the borrelia becomes inaccessible to antibiotics. In the case of disease, only an immune booster suited to the person on a strictly individual basis can promise success in overcoming the debility.

The international literature on the treatment of Lyme disease exhausts itself in discussion of the variations in chemotherapeutic dosing, symptom suppression, and morphic alterations. Frequently, in spite of "successful" antibiotic treatment, a secondary disease picture will be described. Called *Post Lyme Syndrome*, this offers no further help to the patient. The powerlessness of allopathic medicine in the face of the Lyme phenomenon culminates in frank admissions such as the following: "New discoveries by Steere, the American Lyme disease expert, show that among a portion of the patients cured (!) by antibiotics, the complaints resultant upon auto-immune processes continue to exist wholly or in part."

Prevention Using Homeopathy

Among homeopaths internationally there are two schools. The one is of the opinion that homeopathy in principle is first and foremost a therapeutic method that can never work prophylactically. The other school points to the good results which homeopathic treatment has achieved in epidemic outbreaks from Hahnemann's time till our own, winning for homeopathy a place in the spectrum of preventive measures.

In the years from 1799 to 1801, when Hahnemann lived in Koenigslutter, an epidemic of scarlet fever raged. In contrast to present times, poor nutrition and hygiene made scarlet fever a dangerous disease with a death rate approaching 35%. Hahnemann observed that people whom he had previously treated for other diseases with *Belladonna* (in high potency), remained uninfected, even if their entire family became sick.

I concluded [he wrote], *that a remedy which can alleviate a disease at its beginning, must serve as the preventative means, and in the correctness of my decision I take strength from the following incident. Some weeks previously three children of one family had fallen victim to a very severe scarlet fever. Only the eldest, who had required Belladonna for an external sore on her finger joint, — only this one to my amazement did not succumb to the fever. Unnoticed by those others in the town who were preoccupied with the encompassing grimness, she was the first to show the way.*

This incident confirmed my notion according to the evidence...

For evidence that scarlet fever prophylaxis using *Belladonna* was actually efficacious, we need not rely solely upon Hahnemann's outstanding cases. There are also official records. In 1825 the eminent professor Hufeland, in an article entitled *The Prophylactic Effect of Belladonna*, mentioned some of these. In 1838 the Prussian authorities demanded that their doctors use *Belladonna* preventively during a scarlet fever epidemic occurrence, as threatening then as it is today. Unfortunately, academics today regard Hufeland as only a name. Against his unbiased frankness in testifying to the reality of nature and the experience of practice are opposed pseudo-scientific dogmatism and the intercession of commercial interests.

Samuel Hahnemann practised as a doctor in Koethen from 1830 to 1831. During this time, Asiatic cholera, a previously unknown epidemic stemming from eastern Europe, advanced into Germany. In several publications Hahnemann determined the illness profile, and thus the typical, characteristic symptoms that accompanied cholera. Using the homeopathic procedure, he sought *from the store of medicines known precisely for their effects*, the remedy which was most similar to the overall array of symptoms. This turned out to be camphor. Though it was at that time still in an unpotentized form, Hahnemann used camphor to treat all of his patients, even advising them to carry a piece of camphor about on their person. Of the more than 1,000 individuals whom Hahnemann thus cared for preventively, only a handful became sick, even though the morbidity rate in the afflicted regions otherwise lay around 50%.

Recent experiences have been reported in connection with the outbreaks of plague in India in the 1990s, where homeopaths with their therapeutic and preventive measures proved more rapid and much more successful than allopathic physicians in stemming the contagion, such that the Indian government decided henceforth to enlist homeopathic physicians as a first line of defense against that disease.

The experiences of this author regarding the homeopathic prevention of infectious diseases are very encouraging. Concerning the prevention of Lyme disease following a tick bite we can claim a full 15 years' experience. In this whole period not one patient under prophylactic treatment has developed the disease. However, it is not unusual for several years to pass between the infection through a tick bite and the onset of Lyme-like symptoms, so that a few year's observations are still necessary, in order to make conclusive claims.

In order to understand how homeopathic prevention can work, one must first understand how homeopathic remedies themselves work, and how a disease originates.

Figure 1.

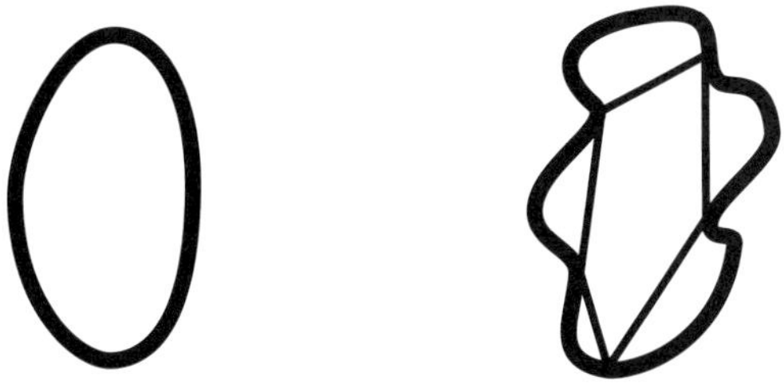

Harmonic field = healthy organism | disharmonic field = sick organism

The illustration above represents the energy field of a healthy human organism. As a form it is harmonious, strongly developed and shows no distortions. (By "field" is meant, not a physical entity, but the morphogenetic dimension, a phenomenon that is technically not measurable, but which serves as a carrier of information. Hahnemann called this the *life force.)*

To the right of Figure 1 we see an organism whose life force is mistuned, which is how Hahnemann defined what it means to be sick. At certain points the field appears depleted, distorted or blurred. These points we may take as symptoms of disease. As a rule symptoms become perceptible much earlier than organic alterations, which can be discerned and measured in objective terms. When it involves measurable organic alternations, the disturbance has already reached an advanced stage. Such alterations are thus of a secondary nature, following as it were upon the field falling out of tune. (Mistunement can be compared to interference in an electrical wave-form, producing a change in frequency.) From this viewpoint, materialistic medicine concerns itself in most cases only with secondary manifestations, as much in diagnosis as in treatment. When it comes to fostering natural healing processes, it has very little to say.

Figure 2.

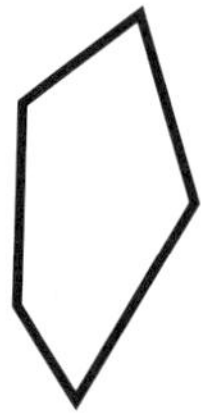

Schematic representation of the specific disturbance pattern of a sick organism (not a disease!)

As homeopaths we take all that is reported by the patient along with the perceived symptoms, in order to obtain a picture, such as is represented schematically in Figure 2. This picture only says something in connection with the disease picture — which is to say, our homeopathic remedy pictures, on which our subject is grounded. A well-trained homeopath, by knowing the overall symptom picture in its physical, emotional, mental and spiritual aspects, recognizes thereby what remedy is indicated for the patient.

Figure 3.

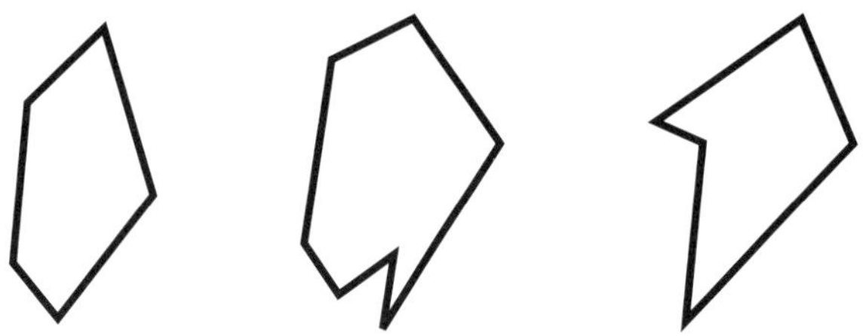

Arsenicum album Nux vomica Ledum palustre

Again using a schematic model, Figure 3 presents the images of three known remedies: *Arsenicum album, Nux vomica* and *Ledum palustre*. (In light of what has been said above, these images should be properly in 4-dimensions, which however is not easily represented. As can be readily appreciated, the remedy picture of *Arsenicum album* closely resembles the picture of the organism with the mistuned field in Figure 1. Thus it represents the homeopathic means of cure.

Figure 4.

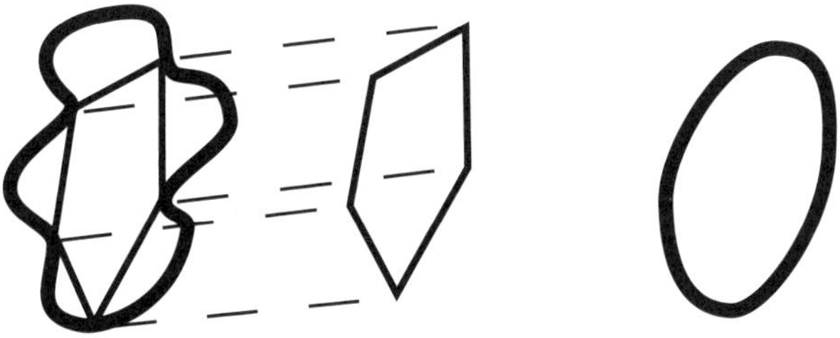

Arsenicum patient with an individually specified dynamic mistunement	Arsenicum album (Information from the remedy)	healthy/healed person free from dynamic mistunements

What happens when we superimpose on the *Arsenicum album* patient, the medicinal *Arsencum album* (arsenic) in homeopathic potency (hence not the substance, but the essence of arsenic, a massless quantum of information)? As in physics, when two waves of equivalent or very similar frequency merge, the same information or patterning in both is extinguished. As the impact of the arsenic recedes so do the previous symptoms of arsenic sickness. In this way healing takes place.

In the context of prevention, we simply reverse the above principle by impressing upon the healthy organism information in a subtle form which it otherwise lacks. As with Hahnemann during the cholera epidemic, we do so by providing remedies to persons at risk (in the present case, those bitten by a tick.) Such remedies evince a drug picture similar to that of the characteristic Lyme symptom profile. *Ledum palustre* (Labrador tea) is, for example, a remedy which Samuel Hahnemann introduced into our homeopathic kit around the beginning of the 19th century. It cured pains arising from joint inflammation, as well as the consequences of insect stings and the bites of poisonous creatures. Thus it appeared predestined to serve as a preventative remedy that could protect against Lyme disease.

By providing knowledge of *Ledum* to those afflicted by ticks, the infection ceases to be bound up with the knowledge of *borreliosis* (which presents a quite similar mistunement of the life force, and which is thus of the same frequency.) As described above, what takes place is a neutralization of both frequencies, insofar as they resemble each other, so that the case does not advance to the sickness stage.

Here again we are obliged to recognize that the infection is not of a material, but a semiotic nature. The Lyme bacteria are the material correlate of the infectious disease, but they are not the disease itself.

The Lyme nosode is produced from a bacterial culture of *Borrelia burgdorferi*. Nosodes often prove useful, when infectious diseases fasten themselves upon the constitution of the patient, regardless of prevailing weaknesses.

There is need for applied research to determine if this likewise pertains to Lyme disease. The homeopathic proving of the Lyme nosode has not been concluded to this investigator's satisfaction, so that we are not yet able to make any conclusive assertions. However, therapeutic interventions using the Lyme nosode along isopathic lines have to our knowledge yielded very few cures.

Until more accurate evidence becomes available, for the prevention of Lyme disease following a tick bite we recommend the following provisions:

1. The tick should be immediately removed in its entirety. As an aid to hikers and dog-lovers there are tick-pliers readily available at the drug store or at the veterinarian's. These serve the purpose better than tweezers or one's fingernails, which can tear the head off and as a consequence do nothing to prevent the infection.
2. On the day of the bite and for two subsequent days the recommendation is to take one or two doses of just one globule of *Ledum palustre* C30. This can be obtained in the first-aid section of any good homeopathic pharmacy.
3. Just to be sure, we give just one globule of the *Aurum arsenicosum* C200 on the sixth and twelfth day following the bite.

A number of colleagues have told me that in past seven years they have cared for more than a dozen tick bite victims using this or a very similar method, and that no case has proceeded to a clinical manifestation of Lyme disease. Nor did it show up when a serum test was made.

Whoever suffers more than three bites per season should have stored enough information in their field not to have to repeat the procedure. One is expressly cautioned not to repeat the preventative dose frequently or at short intervals. There is always the danger that a homeopathic proving will be precipitated, where symptoms — thankfully reversible — of that same remedy can appear. For this reason, the layperson is advised to discuss the subject of repeated preventative doses with a competent homeopath.

Homeopathic Principles in the Treatment of Lyme Disease

The treatment of patients with Lyme disease is generally no different from the homeopathic treatment of other chronic conditions. As always in homeopathy, the law of similars is fundamental.

The homeopathic treatment of chronic diseases requires a thoroughgoing training over many years, preferably in a teaching institution that subscribes to the highest possible standards. Lay practitioners or therapists who lack homeopathic qualifications are advised against attempting self-treatment with potentized remedies bought over the counter. Under some circumstances harm may ensue. Also, precious time is lost which could be better used in proper homeopathic therapy. How these remedies are applied in individual cases is the subject of the case reports in Part 3.

Actually, it depends upon the therapist's capabilities and experiences, just how fast and how completely a cure comes about. Generally, with regards to the skin and joint forms a cure may be regarded as rapid and long lasting. Concerning the neurological form, as with all such disturbances, the prognosis depends on how much tissue degeneration has taken place in the central nervous system. If there is irreparable damage, then homeopathic treatment can only palliate. Till now we have had no experience with debilitated cases such as these.

Some homeopaths are of the opinion that it is not worth their while to concern themselves with the Lyme phenomenon, since the entire focus of homeopathic treatment should be upon the single individual, whose characteristic and peculiar signs and symptoms alone are of interest. Arrayed against this view is the fact that in Germany, given present trends, there will be in a few years more than one million persons infected with *borrelia*, many of whom will suffer incapacitating afflictions. We see ourselves confronted with the prospect of a creeping yet almost unopposable spread of this infection. As with Hahnemann in 1830, who at the approach of cholera armed himself for the fight with preventative means, so should we homeopaths of today arm ourselves in the fight against this modern plague. We should examine our books for suitable remedies, or explore new ones that appear promising, such that in every instance we can cure in a rapid, gentle, safe and permanent fashion.

For the moment it would seem a good idea to look for general similarities between the Lyme phenomenon and the healing remedies that are already known to us. In his article on *Ledum* (see Case 1 below), Bill Gray points to the remarkable fact that *Ledum* is not only our principal remedy for insect stings and animal bites, but it is also a specific for certain kinds of arthritis. Eventually the entire rubric *GENERALS, wounds, bites* will have to be reviewed for remedies that apply to Lyme disease. This approach will at any rate point us towards an effective treatment, as long as we don't encounter indications during the homeopathic case-taking that the immune system is seriously undermined, making it an easy prey to bouts of infection.

The point can be taken further in connection with insects or spiders. Insofar as these play a role as *borrelia* vectors, they may be considered among the remedies one chooses. In one case of neuroborreliosis, I witnessed *Theridion* (a spider remedy) effect a progressive improvement over a period of some months. There are synergistic factors involved in homeopathic treatment. On the other hand, there are other potentially health-compromising circumstances that are best avoided.

The Miasmatic Aspect

We know from Hahnemann that chronic cases must be treated miasmatically if they are not to relapse time and again. Also, as homeopaths we can't rest satisfied merely in eliminating the effects of disease. We want to know as much as possible about the background situation, in order to "keep harmful diseases away from healthy people," as Hahnemann directed.

In past decades no epidemic has acquired quite the mass character as has Lyme disease, not even AIDS. With AIDS, the at-risk groups, predisposing factors and protective measures are well known. But with Lyme disease, who actually belongs to the at-risk group? Or better, who does *not* belong? More intriguing yet is the question as to whether prevention is even possible. Considering that 30% of all ticks are infected and that a rapid increase in tick bites has been reported, in Germany some authorities estimate that one-quarter million people become infected with *borrelia* every year. Fortunately, most of those infected don't become sick.

Since Hahnemann's time homeopaths have been successful in counteracting endemic diseases with the so-called *genus epidemicus*. But can there even be such a thing in the case of Lyme disease, with its bewildering profusion of symptoms?

In surveying the field for possible remedies, it became clear that many practitioners used the Lyme nosode for prevention and therapy. (Out of ignorance, I myself had previously recommended it for prevention.) But after publishing on the subject of Lyme disease, I received hundred of phone calls and emails reporting frustration and inefficacy in treating the disease with its nosode. For this reason I advise against using it, until it is rigorously proven.

In his preceding discussion, Frans Vermeulen described the family relationship of *Borrelia* to the treponemes which accompany syphilis. This provides a profitable direction for inquiry. For some time there have been reports of Lyme-infected mothers, who pass on to their unborn child certain deformities which resemble those caused by syphilis. This fact alone demonstrates the close similarity between not only the bacteria, but also the diseases themselves. Lyme and syphilis also share in common the fact that they can present in three consecutive stages with long latency periods in between.

In Hahnemannian homeopathy, *Mercury* is the principal remedy for the syphilitic miasm. Consequently homeopaths have tried giving *Mercury* to tick-stricken patients as a therapeutic agent in the chronic form of Lyme disease. Nevertheless, there are significant differences between Lyme disease and syphilis as regards their path of transmission and susceptibility to antibiotics.

These observations recall the attempt made by Harris Coulter, in a book published some twenty years ago, to establish a link between AIDS and syphilis. But for all these similarities and connections, as homeopaths we face the problem that while *Mercury* may indeed represent the specific in the treatment of syphilitic patients, producing complete cures in many cases, when it comes to AIDS or HIV-infection it almost always fails. In the homeopathic sense there is not sufficient similarity, and thus the search continues for remedies that are more appropriate.

It seems likely that for a remedy to be curative for Lyme disease it should have an anti-syphilitic aspect. This is what prompted the suspicion that *Aurum arsenicosum* could be employed as a specific for the Lyme miasm. Although there was no actual proving, it is known that during the 19th-century *Aurum arsenicosum* was taken into the homeopathic armamentarium as a treatment for Syphilis. If our suspicion is correct that this remedy addresses itself to a syphilis-like miasma, then everyone who is treated at the outset with an individualized remedy, and who thereby becomes symptom-free, should receive either *Mercurius* or *Aurum arsenicosum* as a concluding remedy. Otherwise the danger remains that the disease will merely go latent, only to re-emerge years later. I myself experienced this in one case which became symptom-free after treatment with *Lachesis*, yet the complaints (in this case arthritic) nevertheless re-appeared after one or two years. After a dose of *Aurum arsenicosum* they disappeared for good. A conclusive efficacy claim cannot be made, however, without some further years of observation.

Homeopathic Research in Lyme Disease

To verify the status of a remedy as a specific in the treatment of Lyme disease requires a close investigation of its homeopathicity both through provings and through clinical experience. In 2003 the Saxon homeopaths began this undertaking with a culture of *Borrelia burgdorferi*. Unfortunately the original material was not properly isolated, so it was decided not to publish the proving results. As representatives of the Hahnemannian tradition we really had no choice in the matter. Section 264 of the *Organon* states clearly and unambiguously that "The true practitioner must have in full strength the purest remedies at hand, in order to rely upon their healing power, and he himself must attest to their purity."

Hence, to the great disappointment of all involved it became evident that the *Borrelia* proving would have to be repeated. Regrettably it was not possible to accomplish this prior to the publication deadline. From past experience, the work involved in a homeopathic proving demands at least half-a-year from beginning to end, so that we shall have to postpone such for a future edition. In the interval it can be said that our proving produced some of the same symptoms compiled as Lyme characteristics by Frans Vermeulen above.

In the meantime a colleague from the *Clemens von Boenninghausen Homeopathic Society* had proved the second "chief suspect," the *Ixodes rizinus* tick, in homeopathic potency. Unfortunately that proving has not yet been published.

Through my own clinical experience I had finally come to the conclusion that *Aurum arsenicosum* — a remedy which I otherwise seldom encountered — demonstrated its healing capability with striking frequency in cases of Lyme disease. Since there was no proving to speak of in the literature, the Saxon homeopaths proved the remedy together. Their proving narratives, edited and organized according to the customary categories, are found in Part 2 below.

Aurum arsenicosum

In regards to the syphilitic miasm, a case from my own practice provided a key learning experience (see Case 15 below.) A very active 70-year old was suffering from the arthritic form of Lyme disease. A colleague who was experienced in miasmatic prescribing treated him anti-syphilitically with a variety of remedies over many months, but without any improvement in his knee complaints. As an expression of ultimate despair the homeopath wanted to give the recommended antibiotic another try. At this point I prescribed one dose of *Aurum arsenicosum*.

Six weeks later the patient wrote to say that he had climbed a mountain 4,000 metres in height, without experiencing any knee problems. His symptom-free state continued for another 2 years. From this I concluded that *Aurum arsenicosum*, more than *Mercurius*, could serve as the indicated remedy for chronic Lyme disease. The additional experience of about a dozen cured cases only confirmed my original hunch.

The more radical assertion that *Aurum arsenicosum* might serve as a specific for a provisionally-designated "Lyme miasm" was strengthened by this same case, which failed to improve when treated anti-miasmatically according to conventional healing precepts. As always, when it comes to this subject there is likely to be some spirited discussion among homeopaths, some of whom would like to dispense with the notion of "miasm" altogether. As members of a wider medico-scientific community, they find the term anachronistic and frankly even embarrassing, in the sense that it cannot be defined by weight or measure in quantitative terms. Other colleagues, in defiance of the materialist worldview, proudly espouse their old-fashioned vitalism. Taking the vital force as a defining property of sentient beings, they have no difficulty conceiving of the miasm as a trans-generational collective mistuning that may be transmitted via morphogenetic pathways.

Of course, numerous confirmations supported by case observations will be needed to demonstrate the merit of this hypothesis. I would accordingly invite homeopaths to publish their successful treatments, or at the very least share these with their colleagues, so that we can develop a comprehensive strategy for the homeopathic treatment of chronic Lyme patients in the shortest time possible.

As might be expected, the remedy picture of *Aurum arsenicosum* combines traits from both its metallic components. For this reason it seems useful, following Jan Scholten, to offer a provisional group analysis. And this directs us to certain conclusions pertaining to the social conditions underlying the Lyme epidemic, at least where Germany is concerned.

In his *Homeopathy and the Elements*, Scholten situates the element gold as follows:

Stage 11	*Gold Series*
Holding/Maintaining	Organization/Structure
Protecting/Supplies	Responsible
Possession/Privileged	Serious / Heavy
Enjoyment	King / Power / Land
Sharing	Failure
	Alone/Isolation
	Ripe old age

And for the element *Arsenicum*:

Stage 14	*Iron Series*
Passing on/ Loss	Task/Work/Duty
Bankrupt	Craftwork/ Use
Useless/Superfluous	Perfectionism
Surrender	Routine/ Order
Refusing/Obstinate	Control
	Failure/ Guilt
	Adult
	Village

There are striking parallels here, which go to show how an epidemic disease very much reflects the life situation of the afflicted population. Professional journals abound with articles detailing the troubled state of the German nation. However, ordinary people, who take the time to leaf through a newspaper, can constellate from a few headlines their own up-to-date reports on the condition of things. There is mention of the State with its mounting deficit, struggling to fulfill its welfare commitments. Advertisements promise to augment our pleasure, while the lotteries suggest a new apportionment of wealth. The current government fails in its promise to create an efficient bureaucracy, blaming its failure on the current opposition. On account of the destruction of the traditional family people are becoming alienated — Such an analysis can be sustained at any social level.

If ever there was a textbook case of an *Aurum arsenicosum* social situation, today's Germany is it. That the psychological condition of a group/family/nation can be reflected epidemically and also in the corresponding homeopathic remedies, applies to other pathological conditions, when the causative agent is known and the (group) psychological background of the corresponding remedy is identified.

This explains why other European nations, which have the same burden of ticks, report very few cases of Lyme disease. From Spain and from eastern Europe my colleagues confirm that while Lyme disease is indeed known, it is quite a rare phenomenon. On the other hand, our situation seems to resemble that of the northeastern United States, where Lyme disease is now endemic.

At this point it might be objected that such knowledge is ultimately useless, for as individual homeopaths we cannot influence the bulk of the population. For me personally, it does help to understand the situation in which we find ourselves. It permits me to adopt (and model) a spiritual posture that is arguably healthier than that of the majority of my fellow citizens. According to this view *Borrelia burgdorferi* is not just the agent of sickness. It is also a messenger from the microcosmic realm, which has something to impart. Whoever lives in harmony with the laws of life (these laws being written on this planet by bacteria 2.5 billion years ago) has little to fear. Those who kill the bearer of a (genetically coded) message do not understand the full significance of the problem, at either the individual or social levels. From long-term studies it is known that syphilis (whose emissary, *Treponema pallidum*, easily succumbs to antibiotics) pursues its course through the three stages, regardless of whether it was treated with antibiotics or not. The same phenomenon, known misleadingly as "Post Lyme Syndrome," has been recognized subsequently in the case of borreliosis.

We should have the courage not only to observe the *symptoms* of the disease in question (as Hahnemann did), but also to pay attention to the *context*, by which an epidemic acquires message-value. With its multidimensional, analogical world-picture, homeopathy is in a position to identify such connections and to employ them therapeutically. In this respect mechanistically-oriented medicine has nothing whatsoever to offer.

Conclusions

A cost comparison using a large sample of patients would be desirable and convincing from a statistical point of view. It would also no doubt be of great interest to the health consumer. Unfortunately there is no possibility of accomplishing this, since the insurance firms do not provide figures as to the unit-cost of a cure. A major fault with the current system is that most patients do not realize how much profit they generate for the companies which service them. The majority of chronic Lyme patients spend anywhere from many months to a whole year undergoing pharmaceutical treatment. In many cases, whether as day- or bed-treatment, several thousand dollars will be expended in treatment costs. All too often such treatments prove ineffective.

From the data available to us, as of 2006 a course of homeopathic treatment up to the disappearance of all symptoms in no case cost more than between $250 and $500 per person. Conceivably, on rare occasions there may be certain extended treatments that cost somewhat more. However, these limits need seldom be exceeded.

By themselves, the current regimes of antibiotic doses administered to in-patients may cost many times that, often without any advantage to the patient.

The cases presented below in Part 3 clearly document instances in which Lyme disease has been successfully treated by homeopathy. Certainly, in the view of the contributing therapists, homeopathy has proved itself the method of choice in the treatment of such patients. Since there are so few reports available at this point, we must remain cautious in urging a standard treatment protocol. Nonetheless, judging from all the evidence gathered to date, we can be reasonably certain as to the following points:

1. The procedures described in the section on *Prevention*, where *Ledum* and/or the *Aurum arsenicosum* are employed following an identified tick bite, have so far proven themselves clinically for all the contributors. Over an observation period of fifteen years, among the persons cared for in this way there has not been one single occurrence of Lyme disease, clinically defined.

2. *Aurum arsenicosum* proved itself therapeutically in the majority of the cases that this author managed. In the remedy proving it also manifested many of the characteristic Lyme symptoms. Therefore, it seems to be a specific for Lyme disease, if not for the Lyme miasm itself.
3. The experience of homeopaths over the last 200 years has established the fact that a remedy can not only cure endemic disease, but also serve as the prophylactic of choice, should that disease assume an epidemic form. (Hahnemann for example used *Belladonna* and *Mercurius* for scarlet fever, and *Camphora* for cholera.)
4. When skillfully carried out, the homeopathic treatment (of the sick person, not the disease!) led in all cases to a rapid and permanent improvement, to the point where there was a total freedom from affliction, regardless of whether the joints, the nerves, or other systems were involved. In those cases verified by laboratory measures, it took approximately one year from the onset of treatment for the Lyme antibodies to fall below the accepted threshold.
5. In contrast to antibiotic treatment, which is often accompanied by severe and lasting side effects, these homeopathic treatments led in general to an overall improvement, without new symptoms (i.e. side effects) arising.
6. Last but not least, in all the cases presented here homeopathic treatment was considerably less expensive than its pharmaceutical counterpart. On this score patients and physicians alike should consider having some serious talks with their health insurance firms.

For the homeopath, the profusion of symptoms associated with Lyme disease raises certain questions as to how one may best “rubricize” or apportion the accumulated data. Basically, we can make use of already existing repertory categories, or else we can decide to make new ones. According to the former strategy, potentized remedies, which in at least one instance have brought about a clear amelioration or cure, can be included in the Repertory under the rubric *Lyme disease*. But whether it makes sense to fill up Murphy's proposed rubric *GENERALS, Lyme disease*, remains questionable. Conceivably within a few years this rubric could look like that of *CHEST, tuberculosis*, where something on the order of 200 remedies are to be found, making it useless for identifying a specific curative agent.

It seems more sensible to add specific symptoms to existing rubrics; namely, those which appear in connection with Lyme disease and which disappear in the course of treatment with a specific remedy, provided of course that they have not already been recorded. For example:

MIND, anxiety, about disease, Lyme disease: *Borr., Led.*

VERTIGO, with Lyme disease: *Aur-ar., Lyc.*

VISION, diplopia with Lyme disease: *Lyc.*

EXTREMITIES: inflammation, chronic, joints, tick-bite/Lyme infection, following: *Aur-ar., Kali-s., Lach., Led.*

Some homeopaths are of the opinion that for certain chronic ailments only a circumscribed group of remedies come into play as the curative agent (this being the theory of the so-called key-note remedy). But other experienced teachers and practitioners take the view that any pathology can be cured with any remedy whatsoever, provided that the characteristic signs and symptoms of the illness agree with the profile of that remedy according to the law of similars. Experience teaches, however, that particular constitutional distortions make us more susceptible to certain pathologies than others who don't share the same problem. Here I would like to recall the extremely successful clinical results with, for example, *Carcinosinum* as a specific for ulcerative colitis, or Hahnemann's experience with *Mercurius* as a specific for syphilis.

The predominance of certain remedies used in the cases either cited or discussed is of special interest: *Aurum arsenicosum*, *Aurum muriaticum natronatum*, *Calcarea carbonica*, *Ledum palustre*, and *Lycopodium clavatum*. In rough outline we recognize a commonality amongst all these constitutional types.

The experience related by our colleague Rocco Kirch, citing Ravi Roy, that *Nux vomica* is often needed as a remedy to heal the cramping tendencies of Lyme disease (see Case 7), was not found replicated in the material published here. Unfortunately, the present case studies are too few in number either to support or contradict any conclusive claims on this order.

Finally, there is some need to clarify the bases upon which we observe miasmatic processes. Proceeding from the biological relationship between borrelia bacteria and the spirochetes, which are indicative of syphilis, one can speculate upon the predominantly syphilitic character of Lyme disease. The ravaging destructiveness typical of the syphilitic miasm cannot, however, be observed in the published cases. Functional disturbances, whether of a neurologic or arthritic nature, generally do not involve clearly diagnosable structural changes (whether through X-rays or brain scans.) Thus, not a few Lyme patients are labeled as suspected fakes or hypochondriacs.

Nevertheless, it has been established in some instances that sycotic taints emerged in the primary as well as the subsequent miasmatic case history, in which case *Medorrhinum* became the indicated remedy in the course of treatment. As well, the cancer miasma could be seen as the principal miasm in certain other cases. Every remedy employed had a proven track record as an anti-miasmatic, pointing towards either sycosis or cancer (the gold salts, *Calcarea carbonica*, *Lycopodium*, *Medorrhinum*).

A general conclusion to be drawn from these case presentations is that Lyme disease cannot take root without a certain miasmatic foreshadowing that involves energy depletion. We can see from some of the case studies below that the patients were for all intents and purposes rid of Lyme-related problems, yet could not in the holistic sense be considered entirely *well*.

As a rule, Lyme disease appears as an unfamiliar illness in connection with an existing ailment, either complicating the picture or else existing alongside it (about which see Hahnemann's discussion in the *Organon*). As such, it demands from the homeopathic practitioner (more so even than in other healing disciplines) the most exacting observations and record-keeping:

- When exactly did such-and-such complaints begin?
- Which complaints began at the same time as which others (thus belonging in all likelihood to the same remedy picture)?

- What is there to learn from the patient's biography regarding inherited or acquired miasmatic taints?
- Did other discernible, deleterious influences come into play coincident with the onset of the Lyme condition? (For example, the presence of pulsed high-frequency fields; vaccinations; use of other medicines likely to cause side effects; or poisoning from heavy metals.)

PART 2: *Aurum arsenicosum* – A Proving

Jean-André Chrestien, an early 19th-century French physician, first introduced *Aurum arsenicosum* as a topical remedy in the treatment of syphilis. Until now there has been no homeopathic proving of this mineral substance.

In his book, *Three Pieces of Gold*, the Norwegian homeopath, Terje Wulfsberg, provides a moving description of his experience with the remedy. Asked whether he found *Aurum-ars* helpful in the treatment of Lyme patients, he replied that in his region of Norway Lyme disease was so rare that he had no experience with it.

As a substance gold arsenate is certainly known to chemists, but is seldom used. For this reason there are few instances in the literature regarding its practical applications or its toxic effects. The link between gold-salts (for example, gold sodiumthiomalate) as allopathic medicines in rheumatic diseases alone offers certain hints concerning the Lyme phenomenon. Likewise, nothing is known about the natural conditions that promote the gold/arsenic bond. It is perhaps noteworthy that in the industrial extraction of gold from the tailings of arsenic mines in Canada, gold and arsenic occur intermixed as separate elements.

The present proving was conducted by the members of the *Saxon Conference for Continuing Education in Classical Homeopathy*. The proving period extended from December 2003 to January 2004, though in the case of a few provers the symptoms lasted several weeks longer. The circle proved the 30C and 200C potencies, as prepared by the Homeoden Company. This was a single-blind experiment in which the proving substance was known to the primary investigator, but not to the provers and supervisors. Although placebos were employed, the volunteers who took them all resigned from the project for various reasons.

Each prover took one globule on the first day, two globules on the second day, three on the third day, and four on the next, or until the prover or the supervisor noted a distinctive symptom, at which point the regimen was ended. In no case was it continued beyond four days. The observation period encompassed between three to five weeks, the reason being that the proving substance was sent by post to the supervisors, not all of whom began administering it at the same time. The provers and supervisors were advised not to share their experiences with one another.

The proving protocol was guided by the additional recommendations which Jeremy Sherr made in connection with the model formulated in the *Organon*.

Stemming from the experiences of earlier provings, I selected only qualified and seasoned homeopaths as supervisors. Beginners and laypersons lack an adequate grasp of critical matters, because they have not mastered the art of supervision (= the art of case-taking, but in reverse.) Should their provers react in a subtle manner, well-seasoned supervisors alone can determine among various possibilities, whether the proving substance itself was responsible. On the other hand, laypersons serve admirably as provers. Being conceptually unbiased, they run less risk of embellishing something using homeopathic jargon. At the beginning Samuel Hahnemann himself only used laypersons as provers, and in general we relied upon his insights from this period. Finally, the symptoms were, according to Hahnemann's instruction, taken down "in the precise words of the patient" (in this case those of the prover.)

The data is organized according to the schema introduced by Jeremy Sherr. Thus, "16 : 02 : 10 : 30" indicates that the corresponding symptom developed in prover number 16 on the second day (the first day following the administration of the proving substance), at 10:30 a.m. A minus sign before the number indicates the days prior to the beginning of the actual proving, where the remedy was actually provided to the supervisor and/or the prover. Unlike substances that are defined in chemical and other ways, our remedies begin working at the very moment when the information reaches the receptor site, which in this case is the proving supervisor. These remedies act in just the same way during a homeopathic treatment, where we often discern an initial reaction even before the prescribed remedy has been taken from the shelf. This phenomenon has been known for some time amongst practicing homeopaths and is routinely imparted as part of their training.

The reader who is knowledgeable in cybernetics or information technology will not be surprised at any of this, for it is quite well known that information radiates at the speed of light. Had I myself conformed to a materialistic research protocol (where the substance obviously must first enter the body before its effects can appear), my knowledge of homeopathic research would have possibly remained stunted. Having proved ten different substances over a period of six years, I am certain that this procedure holds merit. I consider it a destruction of valuable data to eliminate from the record any unusual symptoms that the prover experienced before taking the remedy (and which in retrospect clearly fit the remedy picture.)

Since confirmed reductionists reject homeopathy as complete nonsense anyway, I don't think it necessary for us to cater to them out of respect for their materialistic dogmas.

Prover	Potency	Sex	Age	Occupation
2	200C	F	31	Business owner
3	30C	F	23	Homemaker
8	200C	F	29	Dentist
9	30C	M	43	Homeopath
10	200C	M	39	Homeopath
11	30C	M	29	Student
14	30C	F	40	Homeopath

NOTE: The symptoms are recorded in the actual words of the sick person (in this case the prover) according to Hahnemann's direction.

Mind

I was in a better mood than usual, which was cool, but otherwise I got caught up in disturbing thoughts, as for example, when I read something sad in the newspaper, the thoughts were now going round and round …
03 : X : X

Even-tempered, earlier somewhat dreamy, agitated from time to time.
08 : 01: X: X

Friends thought I was acting like I was all was mixed up. That's not how I saw it, but I had the feeling of being spaced out.
08 : 14 : X : X

Had the urge during the group proving to dress in a more feminine way.
08 : 23 : X : X

Am not quite with it today, forever dipping into the paint can and slopping paint all over myself.
03 : 01: X : X

In retrospect the remedy seemed like a protective cover.
08 : X : X : X

Didn't care to talk.
02 : 06 : X : X

Had no urge to talk today, just wanted to sit in the corner and read.
03: 06 : X : X

Had increased feelings of self-esteem [cured symptom].
03 : X : X : X

Intellect

Very organized, got everything done there was to do, without falling into panic.
08 : 02 : X : X

After my shower I forgot to dry my right leg (the very same thing the next day).
08 : 10 : X : X

Emotions

Got on everyone's nerves whenever there was a mood swing. The trigger: was too late for choir, so didn't take the right spot in the chorus for the Christmas oratorio. I found the city very aggressive, after two beers that evening everything improved.
08 : 02 : X : X

Somewhat depressed in mood, but not anywhere as depressed as on Sunday.
08 : 01 : X : X

Cried as I opened a Christmas package from my parents. Otherwise my frame of mind has cleared, the feeling of having an overview on the problems of my partnership, with relatively little emotion. Can imagine that otherwise I would be feeling lonelier during the Christmas season.
08 : 04 : X : X

The depressed mood on the weekend is not so marked as before [cured symptom].
08 : 19 : X : X

My mood is positive and stable, Sunday's depression has not returned [cured symptom].
08 : 23 : X : X

Am in a positive mood and somewhat jittery.
03 : -3 : X : X

I'm feeling super and in high spirits [in spite of the earlier tendency to a depressed mood and low energy — cured symptom].
03 : X : X : X

In retrospect I believe the remedy had a pleasantly stabilizing effect on my mood, which has since diminished.
08 : 21 : X : X

Feelings of anxiety following a dream, which I could get rid of.
08 : 21 : X : X

Reacted quickly with resentment.
09 : X : X : X

Feel somehow bored, am tired and indifferent. Sit the whole day at the computer and play, not once interested in reading (usually very interested).
03 : 05 : X : X

Today I'm indifferent to everything.
03 : 07: X : X

I feel good. I want to go out tonight. Ordinarily I never do this.
03 : 22 : X : X

Dreams

A friend took her life after she fell in love with a married man. The dream may have touched on a personal issue: I was conceived at a time when another woman was expecting a child by my father. My father stayed with my mother and has never seen the other woman and his child since.
08 : 21 : X : X

Dreamed I got up in the morning and wanted to get the sand out of my eyes, but instead I pulled something like a tendon. I could also feel it in my eye, but it was painless — then I woke up.
03 : 05 : X : X

We (my sister, T. and others) go to a village festival, and all of a sudden we are standing in front of four guys. Two of them are holding another tight, while the fourth is beating up the captive one, until he collapses. We simply watched, none of us helped. I was shocked at that and argued with my companions, but we still didn't do anything.
03 : 05 : X : X

... of a coat, something light blue.
03 : 01 : X : X

Sat on a balcony, as if on a moving crane and looked down. A man began accosting a women, who just happened to be riding by on her bike. (The woman was my ex-mother-in-law, but I didn't know the man.) The man told the woman that he took her for his ex-wife of twenty years ago, all in a very reproachful tone. The woman just listened to him, put her bike aside, and locked it to a fence. Slowly the man's tone became aggressive, and I wanted to go down. As he came nearer to her and tried to grab her, I left with her. She knew nothing about the man, he was a total stranger. At a nearby café we met my friend; she said he had been her ex-husband and lo and behold he had replaced her with another woman. I continued with my mother-in-law and we arrived at the top of a mountain. The road had an asphalt surface, but with a 70 degree incline — more like a tarred precipice than a mountain

— I couldn't see what was down below, since the mountain had a convex shape. I had no feelings about this, I was just an observer.
03 : 02 : X : X

With a colleague had to bring something to a shelter. I think it was laundry. We brought it to the kitchen, a girl took it from us and sent us away. We forgot something and wanted to go back to her. It turned into a cellar that was reminiscent of a mortuary. I sent my colleague to the parking lot to get the car, because we had such a strange feeling. At some point I went outside through the back door — it was night. Everybody was somehow on drugs, they were dancing and dressed in black. It was something like a mass. I ran to the parking lot, and when they saw me, they gave pursuit. When I reached the car, I saw that they had grabbed my colleague. They let us go, but put something in our trunk, and continued dancing.
03 : 06 : 04 : 00

I watched a sex movie in which Kermit the frog played a part.
03 : 13 : X : X

I was diving, something held me tight, I had no air.
03 : 13 : X : X

I opened my brother-in-law's (who is actually a vegetarian) fridge; inside there were only dead fish. There was even a little ray-fish, whose dead eyes clearly revealed its death-pangs.
03 : 13 : X : X

Vertigo

Staggering and unsteady on the street, as if I was less reactive and everything was slowed down.
08 : 08 : X : X

Walking in a cold wind triggered a dizzy spell, which slowly lessened in the late afternoon.
08 : 11 : X : X

Dizzy feeling in my head, while dancing at night I had to leave the dance-floor, because I found the vibration of the floor unpleasant. It was okay

when I sat down or held onto something (happened earlier only when I had gone a long time without eating). Feeling of swaying to and fro.
02 : 02 : 22 : 00

A slight dizzy feeling through the whole day, worsening towards evening, while standing had the feeling I was swaying back and forth. Gone, as soon as I sat or lay down.
02 : 05 : X : X

Head

In the evening a slight headache in the forehead, on the right side, pulsating, sudden onset.
08 : 05 : X : X

Headache in the forehead, slow onset, extending to my nose and pressing down on my eyes, worse with dry warm air.
08 : 15 : 18 : 00

During a cold: aching in my forehead while moving.
08 : 17 : X : X

Headache at the end of my period from 11 to 12 o'clock, originating in the cervical vertebrae and extending to the root of my nose, pressing pain, worse upon moving head, came and went slowly.
08 : 25 : 11 : 00

Headaches in the evening, a tense feeling, which extends from the occiput to the inner canthi.
08 : 26 : X : X

A tension headache experienced in the occipital region, rising from the neck, better after a noon-hour nap.
08 : 32 : 14 : 00

Loss of hair, which I otherwise have only when I am psychologically unstable; didn't affect my good mood at all.
03 : 12 : X : X

Around noon my hair "turned to straw" for no apparent reason.
11 : 20 : 12 : 00

Eyes

During my cold a swelling sensation in the eyes, with the need to squinch them; at night a mild lacrimation, none at all during day, no actual swelling of the eyes.
08 : 15 : X : X

Itching of the eyelids, several times in one day, better with rubbing, outer canthi and lids slightly reddened.
02 : 04 : X : X

Slight itching of the eyelids and a feeling of pressure, rubbing helps, persisting the whole day.
02 : 05 : X : X

Feeling of pressure all day in my eyes, feeling as if my eyes were swollen (they are not), less towards evening, better with my hands pressing the eyes.
02 : 06 : X : X

Got up in the morning with pains in my eyes, lasting the entire day and lessening in the evening, a feeling of pressure from the inside out, the right one worse than the left, sensitive to light.
02 : 06 : X : X

The right lower lid twitches continuously, like a tic.
11 : 02 : X : X

Sight

My spatial sense was disturbed, wanted to put the tweezers in the glass, but they fell behind the glass, which happened twice.
08 : 01 : X : X

Ears

Pimple on the left ear above the tragus.
08 : 14 : X : X

A pus-filled pimple on the left ear beneath the tragus (the adrenal acupuncture point) [nodules on ears are a characteristic symptom of Lyme disease].
08 : 15 : X : X

Mild pains in the ears, brief twinge, comes and goes, worse on the left.
08 : 15 : X : X

Two painful pimples on the left ear.
03 : 11 : X : X

Hearing

Have the feeling my hearing is bad, feel a great peace, the feeling of being encapsulated and not having enough concentration for what comes to me from outside.
08 : 14 : X : X

Nose

Right nostril blocked in the morning, not released with irrigation, became better in the course of the day.
08 : 14 : X : X

Sniffles into the early morning hours, my nose free upon getting up, worse again through the day, mild, watery, profuse discharges.
08 : 15 : X : X

Smell

Have the feeling I am more sensitive to odours.
08 : 11 : X : X

Face

Occasional flushing of my face.
09 : X : X : X

Awoke in the morning with the corners of my mouth all cracked.
02 : 27 : X : X

Looked fresher.
03 : X : X : X

Mouth

Feeling in the morning as if I have bad breath, a sort of gastric smell, no more definite than that.
08 : 05 : X : X

Bleeding gums.
08 : 24 : X : X

Through the day the feeling of increasing thirst, as if my mouth was a bit dry.
02 : X : X : X

Taste

Sticky taste.
08 : 16 : X : X

Teeth

A dull pain from the scar where a tooth (28) was pulled.
08 : 04 : X : X

Throat

Cold feeling, as if I had eaten a menthol candy, a humid cold, with a scratch in my throat and a slight cough.
08 : 01 : X : X

Tenacious phlegm in my throat, even worse at night two days ago, hard to bring up, clear white, like a permanent coating in my throat, had to swallow constantly.
09 : 05 : X : X

Phlegm in my throat tastes metallic.
03 : 01 : X : X

Neck

Drawing pain in the neck muscles, right rear, shortly after the sauna.
08 : 01 : X : X

Stomach

Hard getting to sleep, had to get up around 0:30 on account of ravenous hunger, had to eat.
08 : 03 : 00 : 30

Awoke with heartburn, very violent pain as never before experienced, bore no relation to my eating patterns of the day before — ate meat, which I seldom do; persistent cramping pain from my stomach to under my chin, upon taking the remedy it suddenly disappeared [old symptom, but never that intense].
08 : 04 : 07 : 00

Terrible heartburn upon waking in the morning, up to beneath the shoulder blades and under the shoulders after a completely normal meal, awoke from it. The pain extended from beneath my chin and alternated from right to left in my lower abdomen, a dull, crampy pain, which throbbed just a little. When I awoke I lay on my left side and only the right side of my body was in pain. After turning onto my right side the pain extended to both sides. The pain went away 15 minutes after getting up [heartburn is an old symptom, but never that intense].
08 : 07 : X : X

Light heartburn, lasting around 15 minutes, another cramping pain under my breastbone, less often experienced before the proving.
08 : 08 : 20 : 00

Heartburn in the afternoon, a light, dull cramp while lying, better for getting up and for eating.
08 : 22 : X : X

Thirstless during the fever.
08 : 14 : 23 : 00

Was really hungry in the evening and cooked something for myself, but the meal didn't satisfy me, ate again around one o'clock at night, was still not full and went back to sleep hungry, stronger appetite with salivation.
02 : 04 : 01 : 00

The whole day thirsty for cold drinks, usually drink only in the morning and then again in the evening — now all day long.
02 : 04 : X : X

Hungry feeling and an appetite for warm, cooked food, with salivation.
02 : 04 : X : X

Abdomen

Feeling as if my lower abdomen is bloated with gas, with no relief, as is usual before my period.
08 : 09 : 14 : 00

Pain beneath my left ribcage, dull pressure, which suddenly came and went, and lasted about half an hour.
08 : 14 : 21 : 00

Something working in the lower left abdomen, tugging and roiling, as if something was being pummeled.
08 : 16 : 15 : 00

Am still bloated, which is normally over with by the end of my period.
08 : 28 : X : X

Burning in my abdomen, better with the passing of (watery) stools, my abdomen felt sensitive to touch.
09 : 09 : X : X

Pinching in my abdomen below the navel, sudden onset, then an urge to stool and then it's okay, repeatedly pressing my hand into my abdomen, or massage feels good.
02 : 04 : 11 : 00 and 16 : 00 and 21 : 00

Pinching in my abdomen, relatively sudden onset, lessening after stool.
02 : 05 : 16 : 00 and 21 : 00

Pains in the area of my right groin, as if my appendix wanted to pop out. Tolerable when I'm sitting down, as soon as I get up, there's a pressure in my lower abdomen as if everything wanted to fall out.
03 : 01 : 18 : 00

Terrible cramping in my abdomen a half hour after getting up, only slightly better with warmth, doubling up and lying down, worse standing, my abdomen is bloated and full of gas.
10 : 03 : 07 : 00

At night abdomen full and tense, no gas or stool passed.
10 : 05 : X : X

Distended abdomen with a full feeling, morning and night, better after passing stool with some gas.
10 : 11 : X : X

Rectum

Massive diarrhea, running like water, with burning in my abdomen, which improved after stool.
09 : 09 : X : X

Stool

Stool now mostly firm [usually mushy — cured symptom].
08 : 14 : X : X

Urinary System

Stitching pain in the kidney region, again in the early evening, a stitch downwards from above, a fine stitch, rather like a drawing pain?
08 : 02 : 15 : 15

Dull pressure in the kidney region, as if something was working there, came suddenly and quickly went away.
08 : 04 : 02 : 00

Urine

Today my urine is dark and smells sweetish.
03 : 25 : X : X

Male Genitalia

Increased libido.
09 : X : X : X

Female Genitalia

Drawing pain in the lower abdomen, one week after my period, while doing yoga.
08 : 02 : X : X

Metrorrhagia on the 18th day of my cycle, clear flow, later turning dark, the blood smelling sweetish (like baby stools in a diaper), with an empty feeling in my epigastrium.
08 : 11-15 : X : X

A twinge in my left lower abdomen from noon to 3 o'clock and around 6 o'clock, from above downwards into my left pelvis.
08 : 15 : 12 : 00

Have super-punctual periods, interestingly without a trace of the usual abdominal and back-pains for the first 4 days, not the same old back-pains which would go down into my legs [cured symptom].
02 : 08 : 16 : 00

My period came towards 6 p.m. on the 24th day, very strong, but without the usual cramps that would come with such a strong flow, I only felt just a little uptight [cured symptom].
08 : 22 : 18 : 00

Had my period for the first time in two years [cured symptom].
03 : X : X : X

Breast

In the morning my left breast hurt, aching in the front area.
08 : 04 : X : X

Two or three times every half hour, a stitch to the right near my breastbone, a sharp pain, like the prick of a needle.
08 : 01 : 09 : 30

Dull pain in my right breast, deep inside.
08 : 02 : 10 : 00

Stitches all around the entire breastbone.
08 : 01 : 02 : 00

Chilly feeling between my breastbone and my heart, as if I had breathed in cold air, cold and empty, generally at the level of my nipples.
08 : 02 : 22 : 00

Stitching pains in my right breast, at times radiating to the breastbone, at other times radiating to my liver, tiny distinct stitches, lasting 10 to 15 minutes.
08 : 09 : 13 : 00

Pains in my right breast, dull, stitching, deep inside, several times a day.
08 : 20 : X : X

Cough

Coughing at night, triggered by cold air.
08 : 11 : X : X

Coughing from a scratch in my throat.
08 : 15 : X : X

Back

The thoracic vertebra at the level of the lower border of the shoulder blades hurts when pressing on it.
08 : 25 : X : X

Stitching pain in the left iliosacral joint while walking.
08 : 27 : X : X

A pain which has lasted for three days either level with right shoulder blade or right below between the ribs and the shoulder blade, a feeling of pressure, producing a kind of constriction, worse at night, while lying on the painful side, and from pressure on the shoulder blade.
09 : 05 : X : X

Awake from 4 a.m. with pains under my right shoulder blade, absent during the day, no problem going to sleep at night, but then I didn't know about the pains, how I should lie, a pressing, unceasing pain which nothing helped.

While moving during the day it was absent, vanished in the course of the morning, only to return after midnight.
09 : 07 : 04 : 00

Woke this morning with heavy back pains on the left (at the level of the 5th thoracic vertebra), between the backbone and the shoulder blade, worse when I moved my left arm, better when lying down. From there a feeling of weakness radiated to my lower back, making it difficult to keep my body upright.
02 : 05 : X : X

Heavy back pains the whole day, radiating downwards from the pain site near the left shoulder blade, a weakness in my back, which became quite noticeable when I sat up straight.
02 : 06 : X : X

Back pains on the left near my shoulder blade, stitching pain there when moving my arm, better when sitting and lying.
02 : 07 : X : X

After 9 p.m. my back always hurts, have to lay down or sit back, letting up towards bedtime, all right in the morning.
02 : 23 : 21 : 00

Extremities
While working my left shoulder hurt.
08 : 04 : X : X

My right arm was extremely numb after lying on it asleep. Had extreme pain the entire day around my shoulder blades, especially on the right.
03 : 25 : X : X

My right arm hurts like tendonitis, with a feeling of numbness in my fingers, I can hardly move my fingers without pain, which runs to the upper arm, better for warmth and gentle pressure, the right arm is colder than the left.
03 : 15 : X : X

Dull, constricting pain in my left forefoot, lasting 10 minutes, which just as suddenly came as went.
08 : 13 : 10 : 00

Stitching pain in my left wrist joint, continued for a time and then left, linked to the need to relieve my thumb, which didn't help though.
08 : 20 : X : X

After straining myself while turning in bed, brief, stitching pains in the left arm and in the left shoulder with any movement, accompanied by a feeling of tension in the shoulder region.
08 : 31 : X : X

Onset of shoulder pain towards 5:30 a.m., waking me, diminishing after getting up.
09 : 10 : 5 : 30

The area around the tips of my third and fourth toes of my right foot thick and dark red, sensitive, especially when my toes touch the shoes while walking.
09 : 08 : X : X

Little blisters on my hands.
03 : 04 : X : X

My fingers feel numb and swollen, just enough that you can see it.
03 : 06 : X : X

Feet and legs "lazy" while walking, they felt heavy and hard, as if you were wearing stiff socks and shoes.
03 : 07 : 16 : 00

Bruises appearing on my left thigh and right lower leg, veins protruding on the inner side of my right lower leg and itching with the slightest touch.
03 : 17 : X : X

Feeling that my hands don't want to cooperate, as if stiff from frost-bite.
03 : 09 : X : X

My calves feel strange, as if they were going slightly into cramp, like a mild nettle rash.
03 : 17 : X : X

My calves have become thicker, when I attempt a hot-and-cold shower, they immediately cramp up.
03 : 19 : X : X

Hands and feet go to sleep frequently.
03 : X : X : X

Toes repeatedly go to sleep.
03 : 17 : X : X

My feet and legs constantly go to sleep, worse at night, better with the warmth of bed.
03 : X : X : X

Feeling in the muscles (principally my limbs) like a sore muscle, although there was no previous physical activity.
11 : 03 : X : X

Sleep
Bad, frequent waking, light, restless sleep.
08 : 01 : X : X

Woke up twice in the night, around 2 a.m. and around 5:30 a.m., but immediately went back to sleep.
08 : 04 : 02 : 30

Slept poorly, had to get up around 12:30 a.m. due to my voracious appetite, had to eat.
08 : 03 : 00 : 30

Slept very poorly, towards 2 a.m. needed to smoke, practiced piano for another hour at night, usually don't sleep that badly.
08 : 01 : 02 : 00

Woke around 1:30 a.m. and couldn't go back to sleep for some time.
08 : 16 : 01 : 30

Can't go to sleep because of back pain and ocular pressure.
02 : 06 : X : X

Woke early around 5 a.m., really freezing, though I felt I had sweated (like a cold sweat in bed), couldn't go back to sleep right away.
02 : 06 : 05 : 00

Went to sleep while sitting on the angled bench, although I had slept long and well that night.
03 : X : X : X

Very little sleep, simply not tired, awake till midnight or 1 a.m., then a good deep sleep (by 8:30 p.m. I am usually so tired that I have to go to bed) [cured symptom].
03 : X : X : X

Lay awake till 2:30 a.m., went to sleep only with difficulty.
03 : 13 : 02 : 30

Heat / Fever / Chill

Chilly, but the cold doesn't penetrate, frequent goose-bumps.
08 : 01 : 10 : 00

For a few days very warm at night, even too warm (usually fairly chilly).
08 : 11 : X : X

Fever at night with accompanying chilly feeling on my back, followed by sweat.
08 : 14 : 23 : 00

Shivering from cold with vertigo and nausea, temperature 38.5° C.
09 : 10 : X : X

I was always cold, in bed, at home and at work, always becoming worse at night, then I wanted to go to bed.
02 : 31 : X : X

Woke up once in the night with chills, feeling that the bed was damp with sweat, which I usually only experience when I have a fever.
02 : 31 : X : X

A spell of chills, freezing so much that I either really trembled or had the shakes.
03 : 09 : 21 : 00-23 : 00

Sweat

No night sweat, despite heavy meals after 9 p.m. the two previous nights [cured symptom].
08 : 5 : X : X

An altogether terrible night sweat during my period, the bed sheet was really wet, to the point that I had to reverse it several times.
08 : 23 : X : X

Woke early around 5 a.m., really freezing, though I felt I had sweated (like a cold sweat in bed), couldn't go back to sleep right away.
02 : 06 : 05 : 00

Unusually heavy sweat, smelling vinegary and sweet, had to wash constantly.
03 : 10 : X : X

Generals

The left side of my body was tense doing yoga exercises.
08 : 04 : X : X

Somehow I've become immobilized. Everything hurts, as if my tendons were shrinking. Movements and yoga exercises, which I could do effortlessly two weeks ago, now cause pain.
03 : 18 : X : X

Feel completely exhausted and unwell.
02 : 06 : X : X

On the whole my cold is worse at night.
08 : 15 : X : X

Early flu symptoms (tiredness, fatigue, indifference) lasting the whole day.
11: 03 : X : X

Sensitive to draft, when I feel a draft, my nose and eyes immediately swell up, and I also get cold feet.
08 : 16 : X : X

Pronounced distaste for eggs, I even felt sick when I saw a tennis ball.
08 : 22 : X : X

Craving for food that is heavy, fat and sweet.
10 : 03 : X : X

Craving for sweets, which cause a slight discomfort in my stomach.
10 : 03 : 15 : 00

Craving for warm food.
02 : 04 : X : X

Violent craving for coffee, "which I would almost die for..."
05 : 21 : X : X

Pronounced craving for sweets, coffee and alcohol.
10 : 05 : X : X

While going to sleep at night, like an electric shock through my whole body, I jerked and was awake again, but then immediately went back to sleep.
09 : 06 : X : X

In touching my assistant we both got an electric shock.
08 : 02 : 16 : 00

Frequent bouts of the shakes.
03 : X : X : X

Less desire for cigarettes.
03 : 08 : X : X

Eating generally improves my state.
10 : 05 : X : X

Additional third-party circumstances and observations

I received a lot of help, my assistants took over for me, but also from total strangers.
08 : 01 : X : X

Lost a ring on New Year's Eve, which had a certain sentimental value for me. I bought it after coming out of a psychological depression. I lost this ring once before and then bought a new one. This time I can easily let it go. I will not buy another. I am certain that it will be found and that I will get it back, although I don't really want that. [It was actually returned 10 days later.]
08 : 10 : X : X

My wife thinks I am more lovable than usual.
09 : 05 : X : X

Three months after taking the remedy: an unusual fever episode, reaching 41° C within one day, the most awful pains in my limbs, above all in my legs, which were ameliorated only with motion, even in bed I had to be constantly moving my legs. Strong headaches, ameliorated by hanging my head backwards over the bed. [*Rhus toxicodendron* 12C improved the leg pains, but not the headache.] My temperature stayed at 41° C for a whole day, than at 39° C for another day, than 37° C, thereafter as far as possible free of complaints. I had never before experienced anything similar.
09 : 90 : X : X

The prover felt so much better psychologically during the remedy proving, that a few months later she took a further dose of her proving potency (200C). This so much improved her difficult hormonal problems that she in fact became pregnant and is now the mother of a 2-year-old son. These hormone problems resulted from doses of hormones which were given to her as a child, to curtail her growth in height. Until then, even though she had never used birth control, she was unable to conceive. [cured symptom].
09 : X : X : X

In the morning people kept telling me that I had gone through a heavy night, I had the impression that they could tell by the way I looked.
02 : 31 : X : X

My colleagues said I would quickly freak out, not considering the consequences of hitting people between the eyes with my opinions.
03 : 20 : X : X

PART 3: Case Reports

For this work it was decided wherever possible to select cases which were clinically cured for at least one year's time. In accordance with natural law, under the correct homeopathic treatment, long-term afflictions can disappear which bear no direct relationship to Lyme disease. Since we homeopaths take the whole being as the focus for treatment, we never concern ourselves with Lyme disease exclusively. When someone makes an overall advance in the curative direction, we expect lasting improvement in health on all planes.

In contrast to technological medicine, which deals not with humans but with laboratory assays, holistic therapists do not insist upon further laboratory evidence, once there has been obvious healing with lasting freedom from suffering. To us it is neither reasonable nor necessary to go around subjecting healthy people to testing procedures, merely to demonstrate something or other to this person or that. Therefore only in a few cases do we have laboratory findings available following a successful cure. Former patients may choose to have blood tests out of their own curiosity or for pressing medical reasons that develop later.

In the contemporary homeopathic literature one encounters examples of cured Lyme cases on a regular basis. Often it was not the Lyme disease itself which was the single or chief complaint, so that these cases are not published explicitly under this rubric. One such case is to be found, for example, in Marco W. Riefer's *The Remedy Picture of Candida albicans* .

In 1994, Bill Gray, a homeopathic doctor practising in Saratoga, California, published two short case histories entitled *Ledum palustre* in the British journal, *The Homeopath*. The first of these illustrates quite vividly the essence of Ledum as a remedy, which in fact plays a major role in the prevention and treatment of Lyme disease. The other recounts a case cured of this disease.

In that same year the *New England Journal of Homeopathy* dedicated a portion of its first volume to the issue of Lyme disease. Of the several cured cases which it published, those by Howard Fine and Beth Rotundo are reproduced here. The other twelve case reports which follow below either appeared in the first edition of this book, or are offered here for the first time.

Case 1

Physician: Bill Gray, Homeopathic doctor, Saratoga, California

Note: Ledum is a remedy that we typically use as a first-aid measure for insect bites. It is also frequently prescribed for arthritis, especially for the gouty form. However, I have not yet found a canonic description of the *Ledum* essence in the literature. In the two cases which follow I was led via key symptoms to prescribe *Ledum*, on account of the amazing similarities between the remedy and the personalities involved. With *Ledum* both had a positive outcome.

Patient: B.W., a homosexual male, 45 years old

Initially B.W. complained of rheumatoid arthritis and spondylitis. In his case something unprecedented happened during the initial case-taking. He paced up and down the consulting room, incensed about the fact that both office doors stood open, even though a sign above one of them asked expressly, "Please close the door." In the four years that I had practised there, I had never known anyone visiting the office even to be aware of the sign! During the case-taking he manifested a picture that in many details resembled *Natrum sulphuricum*. However, the most peculiar symptom was that in the evening he would go to bed with such burning pains in his legs, that he would have to pile crushed ice on them. He was a solitary chap, very fussy, orderly and always made irritable, whenever something unexpected happened. After *Ledum* the arthritis symptoms disappeared remarkably fast. But still more interesting was the fact that his nature calmed down to a considerable extent. He could deal a lot better with disorder, and he became much more tolerant towards those colleagues who didn't bother themselves with rules and procedures.

Case 2

Physician: Bill Gray, Homeopathic doctor, Saratoga, California
Patient: Male chiropractor, 40 years of age

C.D. suffered from Lyme disease. From his youth onwards he feared that he would be crippled by arthritis, and for this reason he was especially anxious about Lyme disease. Three years before coming to my office he had suffered a tick bite, after which developed the typical skin rash and subsequently sero-positive arthritis in all his joints. He tended to be quite solitary and got very worked up as soon as his partner showed any signs of dependency. He was truly hyper-correct and loved orderliness. He wanted everything to go smoothly. Many times he stressed: "I would like to have the environment working for me." By nature he was a frosty person, to the point where his joint pains would improve when he plunged into an ice-cold swimming pool. On account of this key symptom and the similarity to the above case needing *Ledum*, I prescribed *Ledum* for him. For over a year that single dose cured him completely of Lyme disease, and his nature became gentle and more broad-minded.

An interesting connection consists in the fact that *Ledum* is known as a curative agent for insect bites, while Lyme disease is communicated by tick bites.

Basing my judgment on both these cases, I see *Ledum* as closely related to the Sodium and Potassium salts, and even with *Rhus toxicodendron* (despite the amelioration from cold). *Ledum* patients appear absolutely compulsive when it comes to orderliness, especially in regards to efficiency and regulations. Being in control seems to play an important role. When things don't quite go as they expect, they can become very agitated. Although it should be confirmed with a few further cases, I would propose that this remedy be added to the rubric, "fastidious, fussy."

Case 3

Trigeminal Neuralgia and Palpitations from Lyme Disease

Consultation:	April 1996
Physician:	Howard Fine, Naturopathic doctor, Westport, Connecticut
Patient:	Female registered nurse, 24 years old

Much of homeopathy's early success resulted from its treatment of infectious, epidemic diseases. Diseases such as cholera and typhoid fever were often fatal under allopathic care, but many cases under homeopathic treatment survived. As a result of this, the English Parliament passed a decree that mandated a Homeopathic Physician always be included in the care of the Royal Family.

The Lyme case I would like to present is that of a 24 year-old registered nurse. She had started getting tired and achy the previous October; but then in January, she began having shooting pains on the left side of her head, in the jaw area, behind the ear and in the temple. After the sharp pain, she was left with a numb, pins and needles sensation. The pain was somewhat better with pressure, and was much worse from light. She would feel very warm, with a flushed face and neck, and need to open the windows. An MRI and spinal tap were done, and in March, a Lyme test came back positive. She was started on Doxycycline for a few weeks. They repeated her blood work and she was even more positive, so she was given IV Rocephin. This did not change her symptoms. After the shooting pain she would get blurred vision, sometimes accompanied by dizziness. She was now on Tegretol for the pain which helped some. She also had pains in her hips, knees, fingers and elbows which were worse with motion and better with heat. At times she had very strong heart palpitations, "like my heart is in my throat." She was tired all the time, but managed to work full-time until three weeks ago.

She tended to get bronchitis in the winter, and ragweed allergies in the fall. She was very sensitive to cold weather. She liked to eat ice cream, frozen yogurt and spicy foods. She drooled in her sleep. Her menses were regular. She described herself as laid-back, easy-going, and avoiding conflict with people. She liked to exercise a lot and walk, ski and hike. She read a lot of mysteries. When younger, she was a good, obedient, happy child. Her parents argued a lot, which scared her when she was little, but she came to realize it was just their personalities. She became a nurse so she could help people. She had a strong fear of flying, dreams of being in a plane crash, and some fear of heights. She planned to get married that June.

The symptoms that stood out in this case were the severe left-sided trigeminal neuralgia and the concomitant symptom of very strong heart palpitations. Based on these, as well as the modalities of the pain in the face (worse from light and better from pressure), I prescribed *Spigelia*. Although she had had these symptoms for some time, this was more of an acute prescription, so many of her constitutional symptoms were not taken into account. I used the 30C potency, plussed twice a day, until a significant reaction or up to 5 days. She was still on the Tegretol. The patient called 6 days later to say she still had the pain in her face, at times during the first three days, but now the pains were much better. Her energy and achiness were also better; she was able to work six and a half hours instead of just 4 hours per day. She had no palpitations whatsoever. I suggested she gradually cut down the Tegretol over the next week or so, while continuing the *Spigelia*. She called one week later to say that she had been off the Tegretol now for 2 days without any recurrence of the face pain or the palpitations. I told her to reduce the *Spigelia* to once a day for four to five more days.

Since I hadn't heard from her for the next three weeks or so, I called her. She reported doing very well; no more pain or Tegretol. Here then, is an example of the proper homeopathic remedy addressing an infectious disease. As long as there are individualizing symptoms in a patient, homeopathy can work for virtually any known condition.

Case 4

Lyme with the Desire to Kill

Consultation:	1985
Physician:	Beth Rotundo, Homeopath, Philadelphia, Pennsylvania
Patient:	2-year-old boy

My first encounter with Lyme disease began in 1985 when my oldest son, who was then 2 years old, developed flu-like symptoms of sudden high fever and an intense headache which lasted for days without relief. I have since found this to be a strong symptom of Lyme headache, which does not respond to seemingly well chosen remedies (at this time it was *Belladonna*). Over the next 2 years he suffered joint pain and swelling of each of the extremities. I can remember both of his legs being swollen to three times their normal size and being extremely painful to the touch. My husband and I were forced to carry him everywhere since he was unable to walk during much of that time. The most challenging part, however, was watching our son suffer through so much mental, physical and emotional agony. He was impossible to please and was constantly crying, screaming, hitting, biting, spitting and attacking his baby sister.

We sought help from every specialist in the area, but nobody seemed to have any idea what was wrong with him. Possible diagnoses included: Juvenile Rheumatoid Arthritis, Systemic Lupus or some non-descript auto-immune disease. The doctors wanted to put him on 3 months of continuous I.V. antibiotics, which I refused, since his immune system had already been damaged by a severe reaction to his D.P.T. shot at 18 months. So I began my journey into researching his relentless illness. At that time, I used some acute remedies such as *Bryonia alba, Hepar sulphuricum, Sulphur,* and *Apis mellifica*. They did help for short periods, palliating at best.

It's amazing how inspired a mother can become when forced to watch a suffering child. I was determined to find an answer even though the doctors had given up. I read everything I could and asked questions everywhere I went. Finally, I heard about something called Lyme disease. Though my son had all of the other symptoms associated with Lyme disease, he never developed the rash. Through much research, I found Lyme disease to be in the syphilitic miasm which attacks and destroys joints and organs throughout the body. Usually, after the first attack, the symptoms will suppress themselves and remain dormant in the body for an extended period of time only to resurface at a later time, usually with worse symptoms.

I took this information to the head of Infectious Disease at the area's largest hospital. He had never heard of this disease before. Still, he did agree that all the symptoms did fit my son's case. I then told him about the ELISA test used to diagnose Lyme disease. My son's results came back not only positive, but with the highest levels that doctor has seen to this very day. We were told my son had irreversible damage to his knee and elbow joints and would never be able to walk normally again.

I finally came up with *Mercurius* (200C) as a constitutional remedy for him because he was changeable, chilly, drooling and had a desire to kill. I also learned about the homeopathic remedy *Knee-joint* (12C daily for 2 weeks), from an Indian homeopath which is used to rebuild damaged joints. Within 6 weeks his joint pain and swelling was almost completely gone and he was able to walk on his own for the first time in 2 years. Not only was the change physical, but his whole temperament dramatically improved.

My son recovered completely and has been symptom free for over 11 years. He never received antibiotics for his Lyme disease; he was treated exclusively with homeopathy. Within 1 year of treatment he won first place in his class for the President's Physical Fitness Run and to this day is an amazing athlete without any physical limitations.

As it turns out, the town I live in has one of the highest incidence of Lyme disease in the country. All four of my children have had Lyme. Fortunately, we diagnosed them all early and treated them with homeopathy. None of them have had any recurrence. Luckily for us (and probably uniquely so) many of my town's 2,000 people use homeopathy and there has been much success in treating Lyme disease with homeopathic remedies.

From my experience, if you catch Lyme in the very beginning with the initial onset of symptoms either at the time of the bite, with or without the rash, or within 6 months of when arthritic symptoms develop, you can usually treat the disease with very good success. We have achieved amazing results treating the disease and denying it any further development by using the following routine: First day, *Ledum* 200C once (insect bite, puncture wound is cold and better from cold); second day, *Hypericum* 200C once (nerve injury, trauma); third day, Lyme nosode 30C once daily for 10 days.

I heard about the Lyme nosode from a few veterinarians who had used it with animals and noticed very positive results. I believe this was also published in *Homeopathy Today*. Even though this does not conform to the concept of homeopathy, which is to treat the individual and not the disease, I have recommended this 'routine' to over 100 people and not one of them reported back to me any further development of symptoms. This is very impressive to me and I will continue to treat Lyme disease in this manner.

In more advanced cases I will always begin treatment with the indicated constitutional remedy before the acute. The most common remedies I've used are *Mercurius solubilis*, *Aurum metallicum*, *Phosphorus*, *Staphysagria* and *Thuja occidentalis*. Some of my cases had already been treated with antibiotics prior to seeing me but the remedies were still effective.

Case 5

Consultation:	March 27, 2001
Physician:	Matthias Richter, Naturopathic physician, Berlin, Germany
Patient:	Paul, age 13

Paul's clinical diagnosis stated Lyme disease in its neurological form. The MRI showed inflammatory foci in his brain. Previously in another hospital he was diagnosed with multiple sclerosis, but this proved false in retrospect. In general one should be skeptical of such diagnoses. Many cases like this one (which I experience repeatedly) resemble Lyme disease. In another case a 35 year-old woman had laboured for almost ten years under the diagnosis of multiple sclerosis, until the clinicians found that she didn't have a disease at all and was actually fit as a fiddle. What such assertions mean for patients one can only imagine.

Since 1999, according to his mother's account, Paul was bitten frequently by ticks, without however any erythema migrans ever being remembered. During a boat cruise in the summer of 2000 he suffered a bad sun-burn with acute disturbances of vision, which disappeared again after some time. In October 2000, from a state of apparent health, a remarkable thing happened: Paul developed double vision in his left eye. The condition ceased after four weeks, but the finger/nose test (whereby the patient with eyes closed is to place the index finger on the tip of the nose) pointed to co-ordination difficulties. The clinicians ruled out a tumor for the time being, while a virostatic therapy employed on the suspicion of a herpes infection brought about no change in his condition. His double-sightedness disappeared all by itself. In January 2001 the diagnosis of Lyme disease was made, following which the patient was given high doses of the antibiotic Rocephin intravenously over two weeks' time. That however made no essential changes to the inflammatory foci in his brain.

In my office the following signs and symptoms were uncovered: Paul tends to nap, even when together with his friends, which was not the case before his illness. He suffers under bright light and has to blink more than usual, this being apparent to me in my office with its relatively normal light levels. On inspection his pupils seemed slightly enlarged. Of late his lips have become noticeably more chapped, especially with cracks appearing in the centre of the lower lip. His nose is continuously stuffed up. Last summer he complained of a painful swelling, first on the one nipple then the other, something one sees now and then among children of this age. This can be explained on the basis of hormonal changes. Probably it doesn't link directly with the Lyme infection.

For someone his age Paul is quite small. He fears spiders. He worries that his little sibling could fall under a car. He fears catastrophes and Mad Cow Disease (this last at a time when many people had fear of it.) His mother added that he had a marked sense for order and became very easily disgusted. At school he was attentive to his home-work and at home he was always "nice and sweet."

Biographically it is worth mentioning that Paul learned to walk relatively late. At the age of twelve years he came down with mononucleosis, which according to his mother was quite a serious case. At the age of eight, likewise a rather heavy lung inflammation.

In this case we can resolve upon a treatment for the Lyme disease on the basis of a few select indicators. The above-mentioned newly appearing ones (light sleep, light sensitivity, widened pupils and cracked lips, especially in the middle of the lower one) do not point clearly towards a specific remedy. If we however use the older, so-called "constitutional" symptoms, then we hit upon *Calcarea carbonica*. The mixing together of old, non-specific symptoms with ones belonging to a newly acquired disease provides no way to determine the treatment for a newly appearing chronic infectious disease. Three reasons, however, led me to prescribe *Calcarea* in this case.

Calcarea in the first place does not contradict the current symptoms acquired since the Lyme condition; which is to say, *Calcarea* exhibits an array of symptoms that is close to other indicated remedies. Secondly, I located a Lyme case cured with *Calcarea* in Volume 2 of the Journal *Homoeopathiezeitschrift*, issued in 1994. In this instance the author, Bernd Schuster, presented *Calcarea* as a potentially important Lyme remedy, thus confirming the traditional view, that in certain long-term diseases a group of remedies is used more frequently than the rest (even if not exclusively). Thirdly, a "constitutional" treatment for a pathological terrain can improve a patient to such an extent that he possesses greater resistance to acute and on-going chronic infections. To this extent a chronic homeopathic treatment can be viewed in the sense of a prevention against potential infections, even if this doesn't mean absolute protection against virulent infections.

On March 30, 2001 Paul first received *Sulphur* 200C (according to Boenninghausen's protocol), and ten days later *Calcarea* 10M, two globules in each case. Boenninghausen recommended that in chronic cases, where *Calcarea* is obviously indicated, one can open with a dose of *Sulphur* as a "preparation" for the *Calcarea* to follow. This in his opinion made the second prescription more effective. It should be noted that a subsequent reaction to the *Sulphur* is any case to be expected, which must be assessed on its own merits, and never according to some established scheme.

At the beginning of June, 2001 the particular symptoms occurring with the Lyme disease had disappeared. The finger/nose test was again normal. On this occasion I gave the patient a dose of *Borrelia* nosode D200 as an interim conclusion to the case. His mother was to report immediately any changes in his symptoms.

On September 25, 2002 his mother told me during a follow-up inquiry that everything was great. There were no new symptoms, and Paul was "fit as a fiddle." His mother no longer wanted to carry through with a subsequent clinical exam (MRI and so on).

Comment: In this case, following a dose of a homeopathic remedy, there disappeared certain pronounced or latent symptoms earlier diagnosed as Lyme disease in its neurological form. Nor did they surface again. It is however still far too early to draw any final conclusions. For these we must wait.

Case 6

Consultation:	March 7, 2001
Physician:	Matthias Richter, Naturopathic physician, Berlin, Germany
Patient:	Stefan, 16 years old

Accompanied by his mother, Stefan, 16 years of age, came to see me on March 7, 2001. In August 2000 he had noticed a tick-bite with a slight reddening, though without any erythema migrans. In previous years he had suffered numerous tick-bites, again without erythema. In October

2000 he suddenly began seeing double through his right eye, remarkably only in the afternoon from 4 or 5 until 8 or 9 PM. A duly instituted medical investigation produced the diagnosis of Lyme disease. Doxycycline was administered intravenously over three weeks' time, followed by Rocephin, likewise intravenously over three weeks. While the double vision disappeared, the remaining symptoms, which are widely interpreted as expressions of Lyme disease, did not. These in fact would incline one to the additional diagnosis of chronic fatigue syndrome.

To a striking degree Stefan would tire quickly, and he needed more sleep than in previous years. For no obvious reason he suffered from vague headaches, which began around 4 o'clock and disappeared once more towards evening. In school his ability to concentrate was clearly compromised, to the point where he sometimes found it hard to think about simple factual matters. When it came to sports at school, his stamina and capability were clearly impaired. And not the least of all, Stefan had definitely slackened off in terms of his assurance and point-scores, when it came to sport shooting, which was his great passion. This last fact certainly serves as a fundamental criterion for a successful therapeutic outcome. For an observer might argue that with this age group whatever affects school performance may only have to do with a stage of puberty. But with Stefan's hobby it was surely otherwise, since in this case it remained his passion.

Also mentioned were diffuse pains in the knees and hinge-joints, along with vertigo occasioned by warmth and by standing for a long time. The family history revealed that his grandmother on his mother's side had suffered multiple sclerosis. (Beyond this I do not know whether a prior affliction with multiple sclerosis eventually foreshadows a serious outbreak of Lyme disease in the family. However, it would be interesting to give the matter some serious attention in future work.)

With regards to his life history, Stefan knows only that once he had a serious case of mononucleosis. This made me sit up and take notice, since in a previous Lyme case the same illness had been mentioned in taking the life history, and it likewise was referred to as "serious." Here, as well, there is certainly a need for research as to whether such cases are more than mere chance.

For a homeopath this case represents, as it were, a real treat, for we have here a symptom, which is so peculiar that we can in all confidence treat[3] it as a leading symptom. This concerns the fact that the time modality both for the double vision and for the headaches typically commenced about 4 p.m. only to disappear around 9 p.m.! There is no way of passing over *Lycopodium* in this case. The other symptoms, though not so precisely represented, were likewise covered by *Lycopodium*, such that the considered choice for the first prescription easily presented itself. With reference to the double vision, it did not really sway my decision that this interesting time-modality was not more evident at the time of the case-taking. The headaches alone accorded with the same modality, and there was also the evidence that the underlying disease was not yet healed in spite of the antibiotics. In a chronic disease Hahnemann speaks, furthermore, of pulling out the "most significant elements from the entire sickness history" as an "aid to healing" (§5 Organon, sixth edition.)[4]

Thus, on October 10, 2001, Stefan received a single dose of *Lycopodium clavatum* 200C. Three months later, all of the above-mentioned symptoms were practically gone. Also, with respect to his hobby, sport shooting, Stefan was once more right on target. For some days following the dose of *Lycopodium* there had been a marked aggravation of all symptoms, "as when things were at their worst," yet without the double vision. Afterwards there was steady improvement. As a follow-up remedy he received *Sulphur* 200C. Sulfur fits very well when there remains an assortment of constitutional symptoms, and it functions as probably the most important remedy subsequent to *Lycopodium*, when it is indicated.

On September 25, 2002, Stefan's mother informed me over the telephone that since his homeopathic treatment Stefan had no further

[3] Through the repetition of "treat," an attempt is made to echo an untranslatable pun, by which Richter sets off the German for delicacy (Leckerbissen) against that for tick-bite (Zeckenbiss).

[4] Translators note: In Hahnemann's own words, "It will help the physician to bring about a cure if he can find out the data of the most probable *occasion* of an acute disease, and the most significant factors in the entire history of a protracted wasting sickness, enabling him to find out its *fundamental cause*." See *Organon of the Medical Art*, edited and annotated by Wenda Brewster O'Reilly. Redmond, Washington, Birdcage Books, p. 61.

health problems. Here, as in a previous case, his mother was not willing to bother with a clinical diagnosis. For homeopathic therapy this is also not necessary, since for us the purpose of treatment is overwhelmingly oriented to the manifest symptoms and less to the laboratory findings.

Comment: Subsequently this case involved a rather brief observation period of one and a half years, which in the event of chronic disease is naturally too short to make any absolute claims. Because there was no clinical follow-up, it can be argued that the case lacks convincing evidence. However, I remain optimistic on account of the course of things till now. It is not up to me to muster conclusive proof, because homeopathy has already satisfied that requirement, even with reference to Lyme disease. In the intervening period a whole series of cases have been written up in the homeopathic literature employing acceptable clinical parameters. In these, accurate and individualized treatment has resulted in the disappearance of pathological indicators.

On the basis of my clinical experience to this point, I remain doubtful about the antibiotic treatment of Lyme disease. Most of my Lyme patients developed symptoms and serious sequelae, in spite of early and substantial dosing with antibiotics. In virtually none of my cases have I seen the current position of conventional medicine confirmed, which is that antibiotics are by themselves safe and of unparalleled utility. Others may have had different experiences. At this point I can only present my own.

On the recommendation of my colleagues I went over to administering the *Borrelia* nosode once, or sometimes several times, as the first choice where patients had recently been affected by a tick, who may have had erythema migrans but no other distinctive symptoms, and who suffered from a pronounced fear of disease. I have practised this way for about seven years. Among all of those patients so treated, until now there have been no subsequent developments whatsoever that are typical of Lyme disease.

I myself can remember, within the last 15 years having had an erythema migrans develop three times — once, 15 years ago, even with a hard swelling of the surrounding lymph nodes and an edematous engorgement of the underlying tissue. In all three instances I merely watched and waited, without treating myself specifically, or going for treatment. Even if I would certainly not recommend this procedure to anyone else — just show this to someone sick with Lyme disease! — I must note at this point that until today I have not suffered any Lyme symptoms. This confirms the general experience, that even with erythema migrans, which is taken to be a telltale sign of Lyme disease, there is still no reason to get sick in every case. On the other hand Lyme disease can develop in not a few cases even without a recognizable erythema. In a complementary sense, antibiotics should be used only in such cases as cannot be improved sufficiently through homeopathic treatment. Whether they bring improvement in a particular case remains to be seen. In my own practice this has worked up till now in one case only.

Case 7

Consultation: March 18, 2002
Physician: Rocco Kirch, Naturopathic doctor, Berlin, Germany
Patient: Mrs. K., born November 1976

Family history:
Father: engineer
Mother: high-school teacher, divorced
Mo's side: many cancer cases
Presentation: Lyme disease
Lab results (as of March 7, 2002):
Borrelia IgM (Western blot) — borderline
Borrelia IgG (Western blot) — positive

In the previous winter Mrs. K. had scarlet fever. It was treated homeopathically and disappeared without further problems. Oddly, three unrelated doctors failed to diagnose the scarlet fever, until by this author's order a fourth doctor carried out the indicated blood test, which confirmed my suspicion.

While recovering from the scarlet fever, Mrs. K complained of continuous drawing or stabbing pains in the chest area. She had also such pains around three years before, which were managed by the doctors with various pain and rheumatism medications. Within a half-year they gradually got better, without ever entirely going away, so that she finally discontinued the medication and resigned herself to her condition

The stabbing pains in the chest region extended to her back, then down the right leg to her foot, as in a severe sciatica. These pains, moreover, reached into her neck and head, tensing up her entire body. The pains were worst between three and four in the afternoon, lessening markedly towards evening and in the night. Coldness in any form, whether cold air or water, worsened the pains. Movement eased them to some degree. She suffered nightly from inward disquiet. Her family physician found nothing wrong and wanted to prescribe her rheumatism medication. By this time she had consulted three different specialists, who also found nothing, despite X-ray and magnetic resonance testing. Finally a blood test produced a diagnosis of Lyme disease. Accordingly, she was to be hospitalized as in-patient, in order to get a full dose of antibiotic therapy intravenously. On the basis of earlier experiences with antibiotics, the patient refused.

Mrs. K. came from a middle-class Saxon family. After the Berlin wall came down, she wanted "to drop out." She married and went with her husband to Brandenburg, to a rural "Indian village," where she bought a small farm in order to live an alternative life. She had to do hard physical work, which she found to her liking. Her daughter was born in July 2001.

Though she received many tick bites, there were no problems, and she couldn't remember any details.

The patient was lean like an athlete, 164 cm high, with dark blond, shoulder-length plaited hair, and many little liver spots. Earlier she had a taste for chocolate, which she now on good advice renounces. She really likes to drink coffee with milk. She underwent the complete "DDR vaccination program," without however remembering any reaction, local or otherwise. A very shy person, she presents herself directly only through physical symptoms. She responds to questions in a reserved way, though she is voluble in set expressions. She often says: *... not so bad ... it's okay ... one thing at a time ... the* [doctors] *didn't have a clue ... I'll get through ...*

Though her hands are marked by hard physical labor, on the whole she has a very female persona. Extremely friendly, acquiescent (couldn't it happen to me?), very compassionate, prepared to render aid, self-sacrificial (towards her husband, daughter, neighbors, property and animals); loves reading, especially by herself, but doesn't want to live alone. She dwells a lot on the past, especially around her separation from her parents. Problems irritate her, but she restrains herself, maintaining her composure. Feelings are not outwardly expressed. She likes to be by the ocean, especially the North Sea, because it's not so warm there and she can't bear the direct rays of the sun [*Vertigo, weak circulation*].

Prescription: Borrelia nosode D200, every 3 days, 3 drops in a soup-spoon with water, altogether three doses over three weeks; then report.

Note: Nux vomica in presentation; a constitutional *Natrum muriaticum*; watch for *Carcinosinum* miasmatically.

Analysis: For some time I was myself dwindling away with a Lyme infestation (chest pains for over three years). According to Ravi Roy's experience, one should give the Lyme nosode at the outset, to break up *borrelia's* chain of causation; but should the occasion present itself, a concurrent or subsequent dose of *Nux vomica* (a principal remedy in Lyme disease, especially with cramping tendencies.)

At first I prescribed only the Lyme nosode, in order later to judge the reaction unambiguously.

On account of the cramping tendencies and "poisoning" with *borrelia*, I was drawn to *Nux vomica* as an acute remedy in the narrow sense, particularly when the Lyme symptoms occupied the foreground, while the constitutional symptoms clearly took a back seat. Miasmatically *Carcinosinum* was indicated, without an objective miasmatic dimension being indicated at the time. Above all I considered that the hereditary cancer taint, the fully committed DDR vaccination program, the suppressive antibiotic treatment, and the invasive scarlet fever illness at an adult stage of life — all of which pointed towards cancer, even if the milieu presented itself as Lyme disease.

Considerations: Whitmont describes Lyme disease as a *disease of pollution* (environmental pollution, callous treatment of the natural world, invasive plant cultigens, intensive agriculture with strong pesticide and/or chemical fertilizers, among other things), which only appears on the verge of human habitation, neither in populated areas nor in regions that are thinly occupied. I can substantiate this picture from my own observation. It occurred to me in this connection that in 2001 and 2002 there was a *tick* explosion in the outlying districts surrounding Berlin, particularly where rural towns were developed and built up (with nature being forced into retreat). With Mrs. K. my lurking concerns were confirmed, to the extent that she also lived on the margin of a city, sought an "alternative," remained unconvinced that a sewage system was the way to go, with garbage being buried in the land-site (she kept plastic and glass separate), etc. She lived in conflict with the "Indianophiles," as much as with the townspeople.

Psychologically, I find indicated world-weariness (*Natrum muriaticum*), plus the father/authority conflict in the sense of that she longs to be accepted (*Natrum muriaticum*); miasmatically, the elevation of the will function over that of the self (*Carcinosinum*.)

Follow-up: April 4, 2002, by telephone: On the whole she feels somewhat better, more like herself. The pains are no longer so intense, but the cramping tendencies are as strong as before. They are only prominent in the morning, while at night the inner disquiet has become better. Often she has felt nauseous, as if poisoned, such that in the morning she would rather not have breakfast; but in the evening she feels a need to drink red wine, which relaxes her somewhat.

> *Prescription*: *Nux vomica* LM 60, daily in the evening, 3 drops in one table-spoon, for around four to six weeks.

Follow-up: The nausea and tendency to cramping are completely gone. She is eating on a regular basis again. The desire for red wine is also gone. Mornings, she gets up in a better state. The nightly inner unrest is only felt in her legs. Some pains however have spread. Need for salty things, as earlier in her youth. A visit with her father, who couldn't understand how she could live this way, this leaving her sad upon her return.

> *Prescription*: *Natrum muriaticum* LM 75, 3 drops in 1 tablespoon of water, at night on a daily basis for around 4 to 6 weeks.

Follow-up: July 3, 2002 (by phone): Three days after the first dose she was completely free of complaints. However, her pain symptoms began re-emerging slightly in the third week, especially in the leg; as well, the inner disquiet she experienced at night. As a result she took the remedy morning and evening, which again left her pain-free after one week. Then she became slightly worse, and the remedy was increased to three times daily, which again improved things.

Prescription: Natrum muriaticum LM 150, 3 drops in 1 tablespoon of water, at night on a daily basis for around 4 to 6 weeks.

Follow-up: August 15, 2002 (by telephone): Till now she has been completely free of complaints, with no relapses. In her opinion the remedy helped in other ways too. Her husband said that she was no longer so prudish. She no longer heaped quite so much salt on her food. Without any concrete evidence, she believed that her parents could better understand her. She would like to change something in her life, but doesn't know yet what, or how. After some time she cried again on one occasion, but it was funny that she felt better afterwards. This, however, was something she couldn't expand upon. For one week she had the feeling that after taking the remedy there was no further progress. Even so she wished to continue treatment.

Prescription: Natrum muriaticum LM 180, 3 drops in 1 tablespoon of water, at night on a daily basis for around 8 to 10 weeks. I suggested that she have a blood test done at the earliest opportunity.

Note: Her reactions by the time of the third and fourth follow-up are in full and complete accordance with the natural laws governing treatment with LM potencies.

Follow-up: December 17, 2002: She reported that there was no longer any trace of the symptoms arising from the Lyme condition (pains in the leg and chest.) The last blood test in this regard, taken one week before, was in the normal range, with the Lyme titer falling below the reference value. The doctor was quite astonished, since she hadn't taken any antibiotics.

Henceforth she described symptoms that pertained to constitutional issues, since the acute Lyme symptomatology, which had occupied centre stage, had now disappeared.

Prescription: Sepia LM 150.

Case 8

Consultation:	November 1, 2002
Physician:	Jens Kirchner, Veterinarian and Naturopathic physician, Neubrandenburg, Germany
Patient:	female, 60 years old

The patient says: On account of Lyme disease I had to take antibiotic therapy as a hospital in-patient and I still might try going there again. For the last seven years I have a wandering pain, lightning-like, which stitches or burns in various parts of my body. There's spasm in my leg, hips and shoulder, the right worse than the left. My wrist on the left side was broken in an accident. It's not the joints, it must be the nerves.

[Weather?] I feel best in the summer, cramped up in winter. I am constantly tense and under stress.

[Relationship?] I have been married to a top executive for 37 years. I raised the children all by myself.

I have suffered my whole life under a heavy depression. That is completely gone, now that I am back at home.

[Worst time?] At the age of 13, when my father took off. During my marriage I felt lost and abandoned the whole time. This didn't seem to seriously affect my husband. I always felt that when he left we were forgotten. He went to America for 2 years without telling me in advance. If I had a knife, I would have attacked him. That was in 1991. We had just bought a new house. There I sat for 3 days at the kitchen table, unable to fetch the laundry from the line. [By way of explanation: Her husband wanted to attend the case taking, but I sent him away.] Now he certainly feels closed out.

[Childhood?] I was brought up safe and secure by my grandparents in Mecklenburg. Then we went to some place in the Ruhr. That was terrible. We arrived there. No sooner were we in the house then a young woman came to say that the flat had been rented for her. My father was always having extra-marital affairs.

[Father?] I loved him a lot. He was a gentle man. But I didn't get along with my mother.

[Mother?] She herself had never experienced love, and I didn't like it when she came near me. Father had taken off when I was 13 and didn't communicate again. After that my mother went downhill. Mother was superior to him intellectually and older as well. She let him know that from the beginning, until he turned the tables on her.

At 22 I went to Ireland, because I couldn't put up with it. I felt myself responsible. With my apprentice wages I did what interested me. In Ireland I met my husband. At that time he was very ambitious, very reliable and comfortable with stressful situations. When his parents came to visit, he didn't put himself out.

I always thought I wouldn't make it on my own. In 1975 I returned to Niedersachsen, but never felt good there. Up till 4 years ago I had problems with alcohol and prescription drugs.. [Withdrew all by herself.]

I feel panic in any situation that leave me helpless. I get these sudden attacks, as if green clouds were coming out of me, during my afternoon nap. Perhaps this is because I was born during a bombing attack on Berlin and often had to be roused from my sleep to get to the bunker. I have always had these panic attacks.

[Green clouds?] Between sleeping and waking, when I think, "Better get up, it's enveloping you." I have precognitive dreams.

[Anxiety dreams?] I was on a big ship that sank to halfway up the porthole, then it stopped. A person who is important in my life lay on the floor and everyone just stood around. I needed courage to take responsibility and help him.

[Injured animals?] Just terrible. As long as I can do something, I will. For 7 years until '91 I was a total vegetarian. I ate less and less, and then I had to eat meat again.

I don't feel good, because I know that he's sitting downstairs waiting.

Inwardly I have kept my own counsel and hardened myself. I am not much moved any more by other people. We have three sweet grandchildren, but somehow such things don't affect me much anymore.

[Children?] I had a very close connection to my son, but he was really difficult. At the beginning he cried for hours at a time, at 9 months he had meningitis. He was very stubborn and knew what was best for himself. He created a lot of difficulties, especially during puberty. He wants to impress his father hugely, but he just screws up. He is very sensitive and refined. It's very important for me, how he copes with things.

[Daughter?] She doesn't know how others feel. She lives her life, and only when she needs something, does she call.

[Being alone?] I like it a lot. I don't bother going to events.

[Anxieties?] Sickness! Rats disgust me. A childhood experience — I once picked up a half-dead rat.

[Death?] I sat with my mother, mother-in-law and father-in-law. Those were three positive experiences, without too much suffering, when they went. I would like everything to be in order. It is like going on a trip.

[Rage?] Above all with horses, if they get unruly. With people, when someone starts yelling, I always get quiet, because I won't descend to their level.

[Power?] I absolutely and totally avoid it.

I would choose another man for my husband before I gave up my business career. I don't find this attachment healthy.

[Water?] For nourishment, yes. Otherwise I don't need it. I don't worry about this.

[Fire?] Fascinating, but I respect it.

[Plants?] For me they are part of my world. Trees are just wonderful. They stand there enduring any kind of weather. I can't support their being felled. My favourite tree: Aspen.

[Material?] Wood.

[Crying?] Spontaneously, certainly not. Maybe that is weirdly callous of me. If I do cry, I do it when I'm all alone. The last time was when my best mare gave birth to a dead foal.

[Horses?] Oldenburger breed, which I haven't ridden for two years, don't need to.

[Headaches?] Never.

[Ears?] As a child I had lots of problems, never to recur.

At 34 years of age I had a tonsillectomy. For three whole weeks my tonsils were inflamed. It was terrible, feeling like that with two small kids.

[Teeth?] Just fine.

[Food?] Desires: potatoes, whole-grain bread, butter, eggs, tomatoes, soup.

Avoids noodles.

[Drinks?] Tea, coffee, mineral water.

[Alcohol?] Especially red wine.

[Bladder/kidneys?] I've had the same problem since my youth. I had frequent bladder infections, or kidney colic, that began in Ireland.

[Period?] Over for ten years. I always had a heavy flow, but no pains.

[Nursing?] I didn't like it. I don't enjoy that kind of body contact.

[Sex?] No problem.

[Sweat?] Hardly ever

[Cold tolerance?] I tend to get cold easily. I feel best when it is really hot.

I had a bad riding accident. Two vertebrae were broken and I had whiplash. My equestrian interests left me with all my toes crushed and my left wrist broken. Last summer I had a really bad accident which cracked my skull and paralyzed the right side of my face.

My underlying sense is that I have to be nice and uncomplaining. My mother always said that she could take me anywhere, because I was so well behaved.

[Cancer?] My father had bilateral lung cancer, and my mother, vaginal cancer. I'm scared of it. These pincers paralyze me. [The German word "Krebs" means both cancer and crayfish]. If it could just be called something else ...

[Religion?] No affiliations, but I believe implicitly that there is a power which holds everything together. I try to meditate without much success.

[Patience?] None at all.

[Healing capacity?] Very fast.

[Conversion?] I wouldn't want to.

[What would you ask a fairy if you had 3 wishes?] 1. a comfortable death, 2. likewise for my husband, 3, that people wouldn't do, say, or think bad things.

[Expectations?] To enjoy life pain-free, as it is now, and still have a few nice years with my husband.

[Self-evaluation?] I am rushed, impatient, over-sentimental, generous, helpful and curious about everything.

Explanation of the Choice of Remedy

I didn't repertorize the case, and shall refrain from doing so retroactively.

I first considered the remedy family. The patient's foremost problem lay with the lack of familial security in her childhood and also in her marriage. She distances herself from people, yet holds onto them tight, which is a theme of *Magnesium*. On the other hand she has an extreme empathy for animals and plants, and describes herself as impatient and generous. She does things impulsively and in a rush, "on account of the nerves." Among the Magnesium salts my attention was first directed to *Magnesium phosphoricum*. As characteristics of this remedy most Materia Medicas note:

Neuralgia, sudden, cramping pain, worse with touch and cold.

A symptom that is very descriptive of *Mag-p* is the baby's rejection of the breast due, for example, to a lack of affection on the part of the over-stressed mother. This symptom is complementary to her refusal to breast-feed because she didn't enjoy contact. Since in this case the illness narrative began in childhood, I start with a repetition of the essential trigger, in order to get her self-healing underway.

Prescription: (November 11, 2002) *Magnesium phosphoricum 200C,* 1 x weekly, for 4 weeks.

Follow-up: [January 23, 2003] After two weeks I was distinctly better, and for four weeks I was symptom-free, although in recent days there are pains in my shoulder once more.

[Panic?] Has not returned.

Prescription: *Mag-p.* 1M

Follow-up: [March 13, 2004, telephone query] For my age I'm in excellent health. In the past year there was just one week when I felt bad, but that passed. Please send me another few pellets, which I can keep in reserve.

Follow-up: [January 20, 2005] I wanted to tether a horse and in doing so pulled my arm and "tore" my right shoulder. Otherwise I've been well till now.

Case 9

Physician: Alize Timmerman, Homeopath, The Hague, Netherlands
Patient: 52-year-old man

The patient came on account of extreme exhaustion. His doctor had told him that it was probably due to the fact that his heart wasn't getting enough oxygen. For this he had taken medicine for years, but now he was told that his condition didn't have anything to do with his heart. For all these years his blood-work had not been normal. It had changed in a odd way, the doctor told him, but they could find nothing further. He told me that he can sleep the day away. He can hardly read because he is so tired. He also becomes very nervous and irritable at the sound of loud voices. Sleeping at midday makes him feel even worse. He has terrible headaches, which are worse upon waking. There are pressing pains, which improve with sleep; when he puts something cold on his forehead they improve a bit. Until now no medicine has helped. He complains that he really must lie down at 12 noon, because he is so tired. He has the feeling of being egotistic when he does that, even though it is necessary. He says to himself, "What am I doing, why am I here, I feel so bad," then he has to go back to sleep. He has been feeling bad for 20 years.

It began when he flew to Indonesia to adopt a child. He had many vaccinations, but by the time he arrived in Indonesia, he had the impression that he had landed in hell. There were so many poor, hungry children. He had a strong feeling of injustice. He always wept when he saw children suffering, and he asked himself, "Why, why must it be this way. Things don't work, this world is so corrupt." Right away he becomes tired and gets headaches. In Indonesia he was very sick. In 1981 he became temporarily blind from an eye infection, his hair fell out, and his right arm became paralyzed. (These symptoms very much recall the results of a typhus injection. He had three different viruses as well as Lyme disease, but they couldn't confirm that through the blood work. They confirmed antibodies for paratyphus, Epstein-Barr and Weil´s Disease (*Leptospira icterohaemorrhagiae*). In addition, he had salmonella (paratyphus) and cartelabactus infections.)

In 1997 he thought he had leukemia, but his blood was normal. Yet he had all the symptoms. He had absolutely no energy. His shoulders were completely stiff with heavy pains. Whenever somebody in his circle came down with an infection, he got it too. He immediately gets a high fever and a sort of flu that makes all his bones ache. His memory was impaired. He speaks in a soft and friendly way. He began crying whenever someone spoke to him in a loud voice. He becomes so upset that he wants to beat his head against the wall. Listening to others takes his entire energy, and then he has to lie down. In the morning things are a little better, but he feels extremely sensitive. He sleeps a lot and wakes up freezing. As soon as he sits still, he gets cold. For this reason he doesn't like to go swimming, because he can't get warm again afterwards. He was always sports-oriented, but now sports activities are no longer possible for him. Sometimes he goes walking, but he continuously gets tick-bites. His injuries heal extremely slowly and sometimes he has diarrhea. He doesn't drink very much and he eats when he must. He only eats Dutch food, meaning meat, potatoes and vegetables with some sauce or other. He likes fish. Dislikes cheese, spicy food and various fruit. He is better in the mountains and during dry weather. As a child he had no childhood diseases. Vaccinations gave him no problem.. His mother had tuberculosis three times, and later breast cancer. His blood-work revealed that his eosinophil granulocytes were elevated.

Observations: The man is very friendly and speaks pleasantly. It is obvious that his worldview changed dramatically after his trip to Indonesia. He neither can nor could understand the polarities in this world, how such poverty and such wealth comes about, justice and injustice. He experiences hopelessness. Why are things not portioned out more equally? He changed the direction of his life. Earlier he wanted to help others, especially the poor, but when he recognized that he could do nothing at all to change the situation, he gave up and changed his attitude. That is quite typical for this remedy. The hopelessness and the feeling that I can't do anything about it, things will never change — anyway, no one can help me. He cries whenever he sees children in poverty. At the same time in Indonesia he got an assortment of various serious infections and he hasn't been well since. In the Netherlands he continuously suffered tick bites, and for that reason he can hardly leave the house.

Although the symptoms are clear, it can be observed that we are dealing with the syphilitic miasm. The first thing, which I have often observed among Lyme patients, is an assortment of infections, which make the patients susceptible to tick bites. The second thing I have observed is that the patient carried out a change in his spiritual life-course, choosing in fact a negative course. He has abandoned his hopeful stance — his life-mission was to help and to dedicated himself to others (*Phosphorus*). Having experienced the misery of the world, he developed the feeling that he couldn't follow this path any longer. Right then the parasite entered his life. Both of these influences made him sick.

Prescription: Borrelia 30C

Follow-up: [Two months later] For the first two weeks he was more tired than before and his intestinal complaints became worse. The muscles hurt over his entire body. His headache became more extreme, the pains over his right eye worsened and he had to sleep even more. He had to go to the toilet five times daily and had explosive stools; he lost control over his bowels. The stool was very thin and it passed in small amounts. For two weeks he had a bad taste in his mouth and there were pains that felt as if he were paralyzed. He started sneezing and his nose released a quantity of tough, sticky phlegm. He couldn't blow his nose.

After three weeks his fatigue got much better, he could work in the afternoon and didn't need to take a noon-hour nap anymore. His headaches had disappeared, his concentration distortions became much improved and he feels better when he is active. During his shower and in the cold air he has nosebleeds, but only a few drops. He says that now he wants to go out into the open, where he feels much better. His sensitivity to voices is very much better. He also reports that the stiffness in his arms and shoulders has disappeared. One also sees here a variety of *Arsenicum* symptoms, which appear as acute symptoms, but in reading over the initial consultation, *Phosphorus* emerges very clearly. I was rather impressed by such results within six weeks' time, and I decided to wait. I would also like to mention that *Arsenicum album* is a complementary remedy to the *Borrelia* nosode.

The remedy was given six times in the space of two months and each time the potency was raised from 30C to 31C , 32C, 33C and finally 200C. After a year and nine months I gave him *Phosphorus* LM2, which he has taken for a year. *Phosphorus* led to a complete resolution of his intestinal complaints. With *Phosphorus*, the sleepiness, which still occurred in the afternoon (this was 80% improved by the *Borrelia* nosode) disappeared completely. If he still occasionally becomes sleepy in the afternoon, he himself can repeat the remedy. He took the LM potency for a whole week. Up to now he has done this three times over eighteen months.

Commentary: I have made a little dream proving. I put the *Borrelia* nosode 200C under my pillow. In the night I dreamed of a clown, who was grief-stricken and who knew that he would never get over it.

Commentary by Peter Alex

Although unproved, the *Borrelia* nosode is prescribed quite frequently for Lyme patients. To my knowledge this is the first documented case, where treatment with the nosode led to a distinct improvement of the complaints.

However, it took further remedies — particularly such as have proved themselves in the treatment of vaccinosis — in order to complete the cure. This case again makes clear the above-mentioned connection between the development of Lyme disease and vaccination.

However, I have seen or heard reported many cases of previously treated patients, in which very learned and insightful homeopaths prescribed the nosode uniformly without success.

Case 10

Consultation:	March 18, 1997 (at a time when there was still no mention of the Lyme-associated complaints)
Physician:	Peter Alex, Veterinarian and Naturopathic physician, Wildschütz, Germany
Patient:	Female dental assistant, 37 years old

Family history:

Grandmother:	gout
Grandfather:	diabetes
Mother:	migraine

Comment: Taking my lead from the *Organon*, I make a practice of recording cases "in the actual words of the patient." I provide these same in publication form, with my own questions or clarifications placed in square brackets. Matters that are irrelevant to the identification of the remedy have been edited out.

... I've been suffering from a bacterial urinary tract infection since the beginning of my pregnancy. [*She is in her fifth month.*] During urination I have a drawing pain in the groin area and a stabbing pain in the bladder. For a year I have had a candida infection that causes burning pain in the vagina, along with a whitish discharge and sudden itching. Sometimes I wake at night from the itching. Wetness and heat makes the itching better. Coition makes the pains worse. They get better from washing.

It's hard for me to breath through my nose, and I get short of breath, especially from nervous anticipation or while climbing the stairs. Breathing through my nose gives me sniffles. I have adenoids there, in spite of two operations. From my 10th to my 25th year I had repeated suppurating tonsillitis. Of the childhood diseases I only had German measles. I came down with mumps at the age of seventeen. Back then I was a shy, quiet child, and I preferred to be alone. I read a lot and knitted. I am inclined to depression in the face of unjust treatment. Then I slam the door with a bang and I'm gone. My parents raised me to be ever so polite. I was the eldest of four children and was to accept duties of my own accord. I was very easy to raise. I loved gymnastics. I always kept the best for the end. I liked to make cardboard houses from my own designs. I am considerate of others and keep within my limits.

I was married. Though I couldn't stand the marriage any more, I couldn't get up the courage to leave. I had a platonic relationship with another married man. I always wanted to see it through. I don't like asking people for help, and I don't easily allow myself to trust. [*Her voice and hands are trembling.*] I also don't want praise from others. I only have one close female friend, but otherwise I hardly have any friends at all. I never trust myself enough to get foolish. I like traveling and love thunderstorms. I'm afraid of dogs.

Since my pregnancy I've had food cravings during the night. I often grind my teeth and laugh and cry in my sleep. I sleep either on my right side in the knee/elbow position, or on my back. I dream of people with whom I have a conflict.

I like dancing, reading, sewing and singing. For music I mostly like rock and classical, but towards folk music I have an aversion.

I have itchy skin rashes on my elbows and behind my knees, better at the sea, worse from cold. Mostly my period comes late and I have tearing pains in my womb, which are worse when sitting. During my period I have a tendency to faint. Before and during my period I get nasty headaches. Before my period I feel weak and tired. After coition I get pains, often a feeling of pressure, as if from varicosities, in my upper thigh and in my vagina. It's a jammed-up feeling. Walking and movement makes it better, while standing makes it worse. As a child I was averse to fat foods. I don't like sour pickles, nor do I like coffee. Shortly after mealtimes I often get hungry.

I have an urge to get my life in order, and I am quite rational. I am interested in psychology and esoteric things. I am compulsively tidy and I can be easily insulted. I like listening to other peoples' problems. If a friend calls me for help, I feel obliged to respond. Seemingly trivial gossip irritates me, but I handle it politely.

Now and then I get back pains, which a hard mattress improves.

At the age of fourteen my hair turned grey and a lot fell out. My tongue is coated white. Under the sun I am quite light sensitive and I can sneeze without having a head-cold.

Analysis: The patient first came for treatment on account of complaints that appeared during her pregnancy. The Lyme symptoms played no role at that time, nor were they mentioned. Many symptoms (rational, compulsively tidy, avoidance of consolation, hair loss, enjoys listening to the problems of others, back-pains, better with a hard mattress) appeared at that time to suggest *Natrum muriaticum*. Today I would also have recognized the *Aurum* aspect (dutifulness, compulsiveness), and would probably have prescribed *Aurum muriaticum natronatum*, which is also markedly anti-sycotic. As in the previous case we find mumps in adulthood and recurrent adenoids as indications of a distinct sycotic taint.

Prescription: Natrum muriaticum LM12

Follow-up: I have a fairly heavy, bright-colored discharge. On my fingers I had some raw spots, which have since healed. The eczema has spread on my thigh, right elbow and behind my left knee. While the eczema became worse, the discharge improved and after four days was nearly gone. Now I have an itchy scab on my scalp. There's a ringing in my ears, an old symptom from before. When I'm under stress or pressure I get noises and squeaks in both ears. I have joint pains, and the right ring finger is swollen up. At night I suddenly experience knee pains, which wake me up. I'm awake between three and four in the morning. [*She angles both feet onto the lateral border.*]

Analysis: Some symptoms are a bit better, others unchanged; old symptoms are appearing which once existed at an earlier time; the remedy is thus close, yet not on the button. The patient took *Natrum arsenicosum* LM 6 and later *Carcinosinum* LM 12 with some symptoms improving, but the remedy that fit her overall condition was not yet at hand. This circumstance is due to the fact that back then I still had a great deal to learn.

Follow-up: [April 24, 1998] I'm easily upset. No sooner do I take a quick break, then I begin crying. I cry from self-pity. In my finger joints, on the index and middle fingers I have rheumatic pains, on both sides, but worse on the right. They are swollen. Worse for movement. The skin eczema is gone. I get secretions back in the nasal sinuses and there's mucous in my pharynx. It's viscous, stringy and yellow-green in colour. The whistling tinnitus is still there. During my period I am sad. My feet are always cold. I find housework meaningless.

Note: Here for the time she mentions her joint pains, which will be shown as being connected to her Lyme condition. The patient finds herself in a very difficult family situation which, as Hahnemann already emphasized, can be an obstacle to cure. I decided therefore to administer a remedy to help her cope with the situation first.

Prescription: *Candida albicans* LM 6

Follow-up: [June 11, 1998] Five days after taking the remedy I got headaches that ran from my temple to my jaw, an old symptom. The discharge is gone. The pain in my finger joints is stronger. When someone shakes my hand, I get a severe pain. The left basal thumb joint and the left index finger really hurt. Movement aggravates, and they are swollen. I've had this problem for almost five years. The joints in my feet hurt when I get up in the morning. They were swollen during my pregnancy. From the 12th to the 17th of May, instead of my period I had a brown discharge. I'm in a super state of mind, I can handle a lot and I'm feeling great. I've had some hair loss. The constantly cold feet are not unpleasant. Because of my impeded nasal breathing [*polyps*], I get short of breath and fear suffocation. I suffer from heaviness in my chest.

Note: The improvement on the psychological level confirmed my prescription in retrospect. However, we have not reached the plane where the Lyme disease is situated. Oftentimes with homeopathic treatment we have to use remedy after remedy to work through various problematic layers.

Prescription: *Candida albicans* LM 12

Follow-up: [July 17, 1998] Three days after taking the remedy I had episodes of sneezing, as with an allergic head cold. My period was dark-brown and lasted ten days. I continue to have arthritic pains on both finger joints, the left worse than the right. They are somewhat inflamed. They improve with warmth, but there is a worsening after drinking alcohol and when starting to move. The pain runs from my thumb to the middle finger. I live by the water now and I've had pains ever since. I make a point of stretching the joints, since that relieves the pain. The pains are also better by the sea. My joints are painfully swollen. The joints in my feet are likewise swollen. Generally in all my joints there is continuous pain.

My urine smells strong and looks dark. I have bad breath. Still I have a constant fear of suffocating when breathing through my nose, along with oppression in my chest. I have hair-loss while breast-feeding. Still mucous secretions in the sinuses, and the sounds in my ears are unchanged.

Note: Now is the time to address the patient's chronic physical complaints homeopathically. For this purpose I took the following criteria as characterizing the case:

EXTREMITIES, arthritic pains better for warmth, worse in damp weather — Borax (1)

EXTREMITIES, pains on first movement — *Borax* (1)

HEARING, noises, whistling — *Borax* (1)

GENERALS, sea-air, better from — *Borax* (2)

URINE, smell, sharp — *Borax (3)*

At the time I still lacked knowledge of the connections with the periodic table of the elements, by which the remedy can be identified much more clearly. Surely the patient's weakened self, her insecurity and her strong empathy would have led me directly to the borate salt of sodium, rather than first prescribing two remedies only vaguely similar in their links to sodium.

Prescription: Borax C200

Follow-up: The pain in my hands went away then came back. The pain is somewhat relieved when stretching or pulling the finger. I have white swellings on my finger joints. My urine went on smelling for a whole day, and remained dark; then it went away. My period is going better. The swelling in my foot joints is also better. The tinnitus is still there. The labored breathing likewise, as if the wings of my nose were straining. Mood and energy are even better yet. Some years ago I possibly had Lyme disease, which would occur at the same time as my arthritic complaints (the titer was identified as clearly elevated). That was five years ago.

Prescription: *Borax* LM 6 (ARCANA)
Borax LM 12: September 3, 1998

Follow-up: The complaints have returned. My pains were better for awhile, about three weeks' time. Then they became worse. All my joints hurt after sitting for a long time, and they are much better with movement. The swelling in my foot joints is gone. The ear-noises are perhaps worse, especially when I'm stressed. My breathing problem is better, especially when I'm relaxed. My mood and energy are good. I shrug off insults much to the amazement of the others.

Note: The remedy seems to be working, yet is too weak. From what I know today, I should have used the LM potency from the ARCANA Company at a much higher potency level. Since I didn't know that, I returned to my tried and true C-potencies.

Prescription: *Borax* MK

Follow-up: I went to see an internist. She confirmed that the rheumatic factor IgA is quite elevated, yet the Lyme titer has disappeared. The pains are gone. Often my feet are cold, which keeps me from going to sleep. My energy is fine. Otherwise I have crying jags when there seems no way out of a situation, but that's gone now too. After 35 days I finally got my period, along with headaches. I have a craving for nuts and chocolate. On my legs and buttocks there's a bunch of little liver spots, and also many naevi. The scars itch where these liver spots were surgically removed.

Comment: As in several of the cases above, we observe the sycotic arthritic pains disappear, while at the same time sycotic signs surface on the skin, where they were either previously suppressed or else overlaid by the disease. In any case the progress of the disease is from the inner to the outer, which is a welcome indication of healing process that proceeds according to natural law. This also confirms what Friedrich Graf postulated concerning the mainly sycotic character of arthritic borreliosis. It is not from ignorance that I don't delve into the miasmatic details in their full breadth and depth. Such a concern would lead us too far astray, and for non-homeopaths it is neither easily comprehended not necessary for an understanding of the present data.

Prescription: Borax MK

The Lyme episode finished at this point. Currently Mrs. T. is taking constitutional homeopathic treatment on an occasional basis. In particular, there is need for long-term homeopathic support to help her cope with the heavy familial conflict mentioned above, so that eventually she will gain contentment. For four years she has no joint pains, and otherwise finds herself healthy.

Case 11

Consultation:	June 15, 2000
Physician:	Peter Alex, Veterinarian and Naturopathic physician, Wildschütz, Germany
Patient:	Male dentist, 45 years of age

Family history

Father:	87-years-old, with bowel cancer
Mother:	88-years-old, has rheumatic problems along with a myocarcinoma
Fa's brother:	suicide
Brother:	heavy migraines and hypertension
Siblings:	1 brother and 2 sisters died of typhus during the post-war resettlement

... I've been treated to the max by conventional medicine, and now I'm sick to death of it. Perhaps the cause of my sickness was a tick bite on the right calf, which I got in 1998. In 1999 I had joint pains increasingly in my right elbow and shoulder. Possibly I had over-exerted myself working on my house. I took an anti-inflammatory. But I work with my right hand, and by the summertime in June or July 1999 I had a painful rigidity in my elbow. My arm was put in a cast. They confirmed that I had Lyme disease. I was treated for three months with antibiotics, but after all that the titer had not gone away. From that time my digestive system hasn't worked well. I have variable stools. I imagined the worse, and even got myself hysterical on account of there being cancer in my family. The digestive problems are now improved. But I am still very nervous.

At the beginning of 2000 I once again got increasing joint pains. I have little skin boils, which are probably a sign of Lyme disease. Most recently I got joint pains in the left index finger. Occasionally I suffer from tension headaches, with pains in the right shoulder and elbow radiating into the finger joints — also on the left, for the condition shifts sides. My knees hurt independently of my arms. Mainly I experience pains on the right side, which are worse for climbing stairs and for exertion, primarily in the right elbow and right knee — either the one or the other. They change sides, or they hurt twice as much on the right. They are unrelated to my carrying things. The joint pains are stabbing, as if someone was sticking a needle or a knife into the joint. My fingers are only slightly swollen. Cold makes the pain in my finger joints better. I have an elevated cholesterol count. I first sought help, when I almost couldn't go on.

In 1989 I developed an Achilles' tendon problem on the right side, with the pain focused on the sole of my right heel while walking. But the tests were negative and I stopped the cortisone.

[*Childhood*] I'm a latecomer. My mother developed a myoma during her pregnancy. As a child I got measles and chicken pox. I was twenty-five when I got mumps. I have been vaccinated three times for Hepatitis B, in 1994, 1995 and once again around 1998. I have a big fear of infections.

[*Teeth?*] In my eleventh month I got my first teeth. One tooth has a mercury filling, another a silver/palladium inlay. The nerves are dead on my upper left pre-molars, and the right upper 7th molar is gone.

[*Operations?*] In 1985 I had a wart removed from the back of my right hand. In 1974 a tonsillectomy took place, due to a left-sided peri-tonsillar abscess.

[*Food?*] I like to eat things that are spicy, sour, and salty. Sometimes I have a chocolate bar.

Now and then I get headaches after a long sleep, which improves towards 9 o'clock. I am someone who cannot sit or lie quietly. I sleep on my outstretched right arm on my right side.

[*Dreams?*] I don't remember my dreams.

[*On the right side of his neck there is a brown condyloma.*]

I love the summer. Heat doesn't especially bother me, but lately I've need of thick jackets. I am afraid of high places, especially the Ferris wheel. I don't want to distinguish myself from others. In my work I'm totally pedantic, making no mistakes, which is something I also demand of my assistants. I like to have fun. I have to adjust to different personalities, greeting them with a smile or a sad face. I like to keep moving and at eight o'clock I also go to the pool. I like to put my heart into what I do, for to me no work is too dirty. My wife sometimes says, "You really shouldn't do that," but I set myself goals and that has to happen. I hate desk-work. I can putter about in total peace, treating all patients equally, whether insured or private. I'm not a risk-taker, preferring to seek expertise from my experienced colleagues, or to send difficult cases to a specialist. I'm upset about our daughter, who doesn't really take education seriously. She has to repeat her second year in medical college, and wants to chuck the whole thing in. I get myself upset inside, because my daughter, who has everything, never learned discipline. Insurance salesmen get me upset.

[*Do you have a favourite material in connection with your work?*] For aesthetic reasons I prefer ceramic, but gold inlays hold better ...

Analysis: As we might expect from a dentist, this man is someone who is very accurate with details. But that in itself is not a pathological sign. Only the synthesis of the characteristic signs and symptoms will provide us with a remedy picture. The following signs emerged conspicuously during the examination:

Repertory Rubrics (with the particular weighting of the remedy in parens)

MIND, fear of cancer — *Arsenicum album* (3)

MIND, fear of high places — *Aurum* (1), *Arsenicum album* (1)

MIND, conscientious about trifles — *Arsenicum album* (3), *Aurum* (1)

SKIN, indurations, lumps — *Arsenicum album* (1), *Aurum* (1)

EXTREMITIES, wandering pains in the joints — *Arsenicum album* (2), *Aurum* (3)

GENERALS, sides, right, then left — *Arsenicum album* (1)

GENERALS, complaints following vaccination — *Arsenicum album* (2)

From the literature and from my own clinical experience I knew that, when two chemical elements stand out strongly in the analysis, possibly a chemical combination of these elements may be indicated. (In no event is this to be confused with the so-called "homeopathic complex remedies," those preparations so favoured in Germany where neither the producer nor the therapist ever knows which component actually works.) In this case, however, the mind as well as the physical symptoms pointed clearly to two qualities, that of arsenic and that of gold.

Prescription: *Aurum arsenicosum* C30/C200 on two successive days.

Follow-up: [July 13, 2000] "After taking the remedy I got a strong headache. For 14 days the joint pains were worse; also joints which were not affected before, then the knees and feet. Now the joint pains are 80% better than before I took the remedy."

Comment: Good outcome, the remedy is homeopathic, thus let it work further.

Prescription: With renewed worsening of the complaints, repetition of the remedy in the 200C.

Follow-up: [August 16, 2000] "On July 20 I took the remedy one more time. Everything is altogether better than before the treatment. I don't need any more painkillers. The pain remains to some extent in the right elbow and left index finger. I don't have any more wandering pains. I had pains in my knees after doing some plasterwork, otherwise still a slight pain in my right knee while climbing the stairs. My heel doesn't hurt anymore. The skin boils are gone. Something resembling a wart has appeared on my thumb.

Comment: The remedy fits very well, still a few complaints remaining. The outbreak of warts on the skin appears interesting and noteworthy for further treatment — here the healing reaction has shifted the sycotic manifestations from the joints to the outside, as we might expect in a healing process governed by natural law.

Prescription: *Aurum arsenicosum* MK

Follow-up: [October 19, 2000] I have almost no more joint pains, ordinarily only in the morning and when carrying heavy loads. Sometimes in the course of the day I have stitches and pressure in my heart under the sternum. This happens while resting or at work. Blood pressure and ECG are normal. At present I have a lot of stress and irritation. It's very seldom that I get headaches and I haven't taken any pain relievers in a long time.

Comment: Another disease layer, another symptom picture, is appearing, which evidently is not connected to the Lyme disease. It remains to be observed to what degree the new complaints have to do with the situation (stress and irritation), or else possess their own disease status. On account of the new symptoms and the strongly transparent sycosis in the case taking (mumps as a grown-up, many vaccinations, condylomata, warts removed ...), *Medorrhinum* may be prescribed successfully at a later point.

Subsequent Observation: On account of his habitual thoroughness and his personal interest, the former patient had his blood tested several months later, finding that all indicators regarding Lyme disease and rheumatic factors were negative. This convinced him then and there of our method, such that he undertook a course of study in homeopathy. He has recently undergone homeopathic treatment on the constitutional level, where his underlying miasmatic weakness, which had led to illness, could not be healed in so short a time.

Case 12

Consultation: June 6, 2001
Physician: Peter Alex, Veterinarian and Naturopathic physician, Wildschuetz, Germany
Patient: Male, 45 years of age

Family history

- *Father:* diabetes, gout, heart bypass, high cholesterol, died at 64
- *Pa g'dfather* heart problems
- *Ma g'dmother:* diabetes II, senile dementia
- *Mother:* manic-depressive + schizophrenia since youth
- *Paternal aunt:* severe asthma
- *Sister:* severe asthma
- *Daughter:* myopia, allergies, neurodermatitis (until puberty)

I was a sportsman, who had to give it up two years back and take up marksmanship instead. My father himself taught target shooting. My job is that of a pharmaceutical consultant, though I myself didn't like swallowing pills.

Three years ago I went to a naturopath for the first time on account of an intestinal mycosis. As a child I had an intestinal operation at the age of fourteen.

One night in 1998 my left knee swelled up for the first time. In 1999 it happened again, this time painfully. Lyme disease was diagnosed and I received antibiotics. After that I was apparently free of the disease. Eight weeks ago my hair became very dry and I got a stiff neck, which cracked. I've had pain in my first joints of little fingers since November 2000. There is a disturbed sensation in the ring and little finger of my right hand. Six weeks ago, while jogging, I got pains in my left knee. These became worse after hiking. I received laser treatments, and the swelling became inflamed. It got painful and anti-rheumatics were prescribed. The regular physicians didn't understand my case very well. The Lyme disease is still there.

I've had slight headaches constantly for eight years. After one week they set in permanently. These are especially bad in the morning when I get up, but through the day they become better. The pains lie above my eyes and extend to the back of my head.. Or else they begin in the occiput and stretch either to the left eye or the dental arch on the upper left side. Often my headaches extend to my teeth. At such times I am quite sensitive to light and to sound, while music and sleep makes it better. For years I have had pains in my neck. Before I always thought it was due to smoking. I am worried that my ailments will continue to get worse.

The left knee hurts when I start moving after sitting for a long while. It's a pressing pain. Above the left knee there is a hard swelling. Cooling alleviates the pains. The musculature on upper thigh is wasting away rapidly. The last known tick-bite which I can remember was in 1983 [!] In 1998 I got pains above my left kneecap. It is as if there were a loose piece of bone there. The pains are extreme and unrelenting. I wouldn't wish them on my worst enemy. I get very hot and sweat a lot. Coolness makes it a little better. The place where it hurts is swollen, and over it there is a red spot. I imagine that now my right knee is also starting up.

There is frequent creaking in my cervical vertebrae. Along with that there is a painful sensation around my larynx, which occurred more often before. I always get this in association with my headaches. For five or six years I have had visual disturbances. These begin two hours before the migraine-type headaches, and when driving, always together with tension in the nape of my neck. I can see distinctly in the middle of the field, but I have something like tunnel vision with banks of fog around. It blurs and turns white. It moves like veils and is white or silvered. I have had the migraines for around two months. They begin with visual distortions, after which come the headaches. Sometimes it's like a hair is moving across the visual field. I have been shortsighted since my eighth year.

As a sportsman I led a relatively protected life, though I didn't know it at the time. In 1986 [!] I got pains in both knees for the first time. I got injected with a cartilage-building remedy, and once more it was okay. Since my youth I have had a loud cracking in my knees.

It does my spirit good to go into the mountains. There, funnily, I have no complaints. I would love to run a camp in the mountains and live in nature.

I have read that cracking in the cervical vertebrae is a problem in Lyme disease. Earlier I had a capsular inflammation in the elbow joint, which led to the unpleasant sensation in the ring and little fingers.

[What does stress mean to you?] For me, stress is when I get excited. Even today businesses in the east still have the old DDR[5] way of doing things. I also get stressed with my daughter. She's a hard egg, just like myself. My work is not my calling, and the financial rewards are all that I find appealing. Personally I am in a state of paralysis, but I will not change myself. I get pleasure from sports. I can't help getting upset over my shortcomings. In sports we were always achievement-oriented. These days I see a lot of mediocrity, which I have to ignore. The customer sees me, not the company, and I am not happy that I put myself on the line, while my colleagues are content to do sloppy work. I have to be active, otherwise production lags. That drives me crazy. Flexibility and customer relations are important, but the company doesn't see that. Any economic success is due entirely to the field agents. At times I am troubled that I don't get on with things. I would have loved to become a sports instructor, but that didn't happen because I have nodes on my vocal cords. At times my voice disappears completely,

[5] Translator's note. The former German Democratic Republic.

worse for talking a lot, better from clearing my throat. In 1994 my nasal septum was operated on for a breathing problem. I don't like hearing my voice, and I am shocked when I hear it on the tape recorder.

In 1972 I had an ileum resection that took away one half of the intestine. I have constant wind and a full feeling, often with flatulence. My guts rumble like a juice factory. I like potatoes, garlic, chocolate, fried poultry, and steak. I am averse to tongue and smelly cheese. I can't stand barbequed meat, since it gives me diarrhea and I become nauseous. I get wind from legumes, leeks, and other gas-producing foods. Occasionally, when I'm really angry and upset, I will also get heartburn and acid belching, as is always the case with fruit juices (orange or apple juice). I often get heartburn through stress at work. After my intestinal cleanse I have felt quite fit. My sweat smells much better. My liver values were always elevated, and in fact I have had a fatty liver for a long time.

In 1991 I lost my job and then came down with kidney colic, I passed some small stones. At times I have urination problems and bladder retention. For some time the urine stream has been interrupted.

At thirteen years I had an appendectomy. An adhesion developed as a result, and later I had to have a further bowel operation. Altogether I had three operations. With me wounds heal quite quickly.

I survived a 30-metre fall, and one week later I had tar-like stools. There was bleeding from an intestinal anastomosis, and a little intestinal polyp was removed.

[*What irritates you?*] Sometimes I get a bit out of control and then tend to rant. I can't hide my opinions under a basket; instead I tell people what I think to their face. I'm in a strong position, because I have the best sales' record, and this gives me the right to be that way. I'm no friend of the silent majority, and I cannot accept a wishy-washy attitude. Often enough I found myself beating my head against the wall.

[*Sleep?*] I can't sleep at the full moon. Time-wise I wake towards one o'clock on account of bladder urging. I snore terribly. I sleep deeply, but waken to unusual sounds. Once I dreamt that one of my legs was amputated.

[*Childhood?*] I was a wanted child and was breast-fed for some time. As a child I had chickenpox, and at the age of thirteen I got mumps. I had three older sisters but I was my father's favorite. My father had an illegitimate child, one year older than myself. My parents quarreled endlessly, and my father became very distant. My mother subordinated herself, yet drove my father to the point of rage.

[*Teeth?*] I have gold and mercury fillings. From my earliest years I had carious and crumbling teeth, especially troublesome while serving in the army.

My hair turned grey early on. My blood pressure is slightly high and for 2-3 years I took blood pressure injections. In 1992 I had my last tetanus vaccination. In 1986, following an injury, I had an ankle operation on the right side and another operation on my right elbow. My knee hurts when it is relaxed. Fourteen days ago my left shoulder was partly dislocated, and since then I have been in pain. Ten years ago I dislocated my right arm on one occasion.

[*Hobbies?*] I like everything, but sports especially. Except running — I don't enjoy that. Cross-country skiing, downhill racing, badminton. And I love the mountains.

From 1993 I have had tinnitus, moderately even as child. When it's quiet I hear a humming, sometimes more, sometimes less. It changes sides, but otherwise my hearing is 120%.

On my right thumb I had a big wart that was removed. I have a flaky skin rash on the wings of my nose, my temples, my upper lip, and above my eyebrows. It's scaly like eczema and itches. I've had that from the time it was plastered during my nasal operation.

Analysis: Here, too, the sycotic details leap again to the eye. It is highly probable that his father's infidelity points towards a gonorrheal taint; also the excised condylomata, numerous vaccinations, elevated liver fat values, high blood pressure. As a typical sportsman the patient shows a unconditional will to succeed, which extends to his business life. At that time I had not heard the comments passed on by Rocco Kirch from our teacher, Ravi Roy, concerning the relation between *Nux vomica* and Lyme disease. But I had encountered *Nux vomica* as either the acute or complementary remedy for *Medorrhinum* (a nosode prepared from the pus of gonorrhea patients.)

I also tried objectively to confirm my strong impression of *Nux vomica* via the repertory:

MIND, honest — *Nux vomica* (1)

MIND, ambitious, very — *Nux vomica* (3)

SPEECH & VOICE, lost — *Nux vomica* (2)

ABDOMEN, liver complaints — *Nux vomica* (3)

ABDOMEN, obstruction, ileus — *Nux vomica* (1)

EXTREMITIES, swelling, knee, painful — *Nux vomica* (2)

EXTREMITIES, swelling, knee, white swelling — *Nux vomica* (1)

BLADDER, urination, interrupted stream — *Nux vomica (1)*

Prescription: *Nux vomica* LM 12, 1 x day, 3 drops

Follow-up: [June 26, 2001 by phone] I have the symptoms accompanying a migraine, but without headaches. Since yesterday evening I've had severe vertigo.

Analysis: Initial reaction, a strong effect, the remedy only being taken two days before.

Follow-up: [June 28, 2001] I'm still constantly dizzy. When walking I stagger like a drunk. The dizziness starts after coffee. It's like a blow to the back of my head when I get up.

Analysis: Possibly an over-dose? Stop the remedy for the time being.

Note: In retrospect, while reading the case description, it occurred to me that I should also have advised him to avoid coffee, a measure that I very rarely find necessary. It is just as conceivable that the potency was too low, as I would only later learn from my colleague Rocco Kirch.

Follow-up: [July 3, 2001] My knee pains are improving steadily. I have no headaches. In exchange, though, I have heavy intestinal pains. My legs are as heavy as lead, which is an old symptom.

Analysis: Old symptoms are returning and getting better, which is the appropriate direction of cure. Can the remedy possibly improve things further?

Prescription: *Nux vomica* LM 12, 1 drop from the 2nd glass (on account of the strong reaction to the initial doses.)

Follow-up: [August 30, 2001] I had to give up hiking in the mountains, because of my knees. Now they are better than before. Coolness helps.

I have very thin stools and I'm pretty worn out, like after a marathon. It's worse in the morning. My legs are heavy and I am weak [*old symptom*].

I hardly have any headaches, and my blood pressure is 140/95. I have a huge craving for potatoes and garlic. I dream less than before. The left knee is swollen from edema, but it is pain-free. The cracking in my neck is worse. It's loud when I'm moving. My legs are heavy, as if the battery was dead. Though better, the urine stream is still interrupted. After bending for a long time, the left knee got worse and hurt a lot. It also hurts when I twist it, grating like sand.

Prescription: Nux vomica LM 6

Note: Because of the patient's tremendous sensitivity, and because his problems in the final analysis lay on the physical plane, I decided to decrease the potency. At this point *Ledum* symptoms were also appearing — knee pains, improved with coolness.

Follow-up: [October 25, 2001] In the meantime I've had a breakthrough. I don't have any more knee complaints, or only very seldom. My blood pressure is okay. My left shoulder still hurts when I lie on it and there is a sound, as if sand were inside. My heartburn increased, and I had loud noises in my gut. The pains in my finger joints are gone.

Note: Pains in the left shoulder while lying on it, especially after injuries, the urinary symptoms along with the family history now allowed me to see one level deeper.

Prescription: Medorrhinum MK, 1 globule

Follow-up: [November 6, 2001]. After taking the remedy my knees and all my muscles hurt. I started shivering violently and began turning blue. I came down with a fever of 39.5 C. I have burning pains while urinating and the pressure in my bladder lasts for hours.

Note: A very powerful initial reaction. Knowing his sensitivity to homeopathic remedies, I should have been more conservative in my prescribing. On the whole my suspicions are well confirmed; therefore wait and see what develops.

Follow-up: [November 8, 2001] While urinating my urethra burns like fire. My urethra has been secreting pus. Urination is spasmodic and interrupted. Frequently there is an urging to urination. My urine is dark yellow and smells awfully acidic. I've had fits of coughing along with eye-pains and the feeling that my head would burst. All my joints hurt. The night-sweats have improved a lot.

Analysis: I don't dare try *Medorrhinum* as the acute remedy, although I have had good experiences with it. Moreover, the homeopathic picture of *Capsicum* really struck my attention.

> *Prescription: Capsicum annuum* C30, 1 globule dissolved in water, a teaspoon every thirty minutes.

Follow-up: [December 5, 2001] I have itching further up in my urethra. By day I have frequent urging to urinate. From time to time I get burning and itching while urinating. The stream is interrupted. The left arm hurts at the elbow joint *[an old symptom]*. My sleep is good and I'm quite fit.

> *Prescription: Clematis erecta* C200

Follow-up: [December 12, 2001] At night I have continuous urging, but nothing comes. When it finally did come the urine was dark brown. During the day everything is normal. My bladder fills up quite quickly and I get the feeling that I have to hurry. I have a feeling of tension around my kidneys. During urination I have burning in my urethra and the stream is interrupted. Twenty-five years ago I had inflammation in the kidney [pyelonephrits]. I'm worried that it has to do with my prostate.

> *Prescription: Sulphur* MK

Follow-up: [January 17, 2002] I have a kidney stone on my right side and also a urethral infection. My bladder is unresponsive. The prostate is enlarged. There's a lump in my left testicle causing a drawing pain, possibly from the medical examination. In the right kidney I have a drawing pain when waking in the morning. The left elbow is again extremely painful, stabbing. Worse with movement, lifting, effort. Once I bled briefly from my urethra, painlessly. Urination is better following the bladder examination, but the stream still remains interrupted.

I have an extreme reaction to beef. I get heartburn and stomach-pains. There is full feeling with lots of flatulence.

Follow-up: [April 24, 2002] When sitting the left knee pulls and cracks. The right elbow hurts when lifting things. My intolerance for beef remains. After eating meat I can't get to sleep. The prostate is enlarged. The kidney stone is still there, but causes no pain. The left shoulder was badly dislocated and cracks ever since, as if sand were in there. I have a congenitally degenerating kneecap. Since the elbow problem I get the feeling as if my right hand were numb, worse with grasping and after stopping. The Lyme titer is still there, but on the borderline, around 7 [*positive* is > 9].

Analysis: As the specific symptoms steadily fall away, at the same time some sycotic symptoms emerge, with special emphasis on the predisposition to gout (kidney stones, complaints worse from eating meat, cracking in the joints); so I decided to prescribe for this predisposition — and not by chance is *Ledum* a chief remedy.

Prescription: Ledum LM 6

Follow-up: [September 9, 2002] My overall condition is quite good. After the dose of *Ledum* I had pains for a week, then they left. I took it till August. In my left knee I get a drawing sensation from time to time, but now it's gone. I bicycled 420 km in four days, during which two fingers in my left hand were numb, but that stopped after fourteen days. Now the little finger is seldom numb. Earlier it was more on the right side. I don't have any more headaches. The joints in my left feet hurt for two hours after getting up in the morning, but now that is completely gone. My blood sugar is normal. I have changed my diet and taken off ten kilograms. Mostly the cracking in my joints is still there. Also my cervical vertebrae still crack, but there is no pain. Since discontinuing the *Ledum,* the drawing in my knee has also stopped.

Prescription: Wait.

Follow-up: [October 15, 2002] I have a hard lump between the ribs on my left side. It hurts when I lie on it. The knee rarely hurts.

Prescription: Ledum LM 12

Follow-up: [November 26, 2002] I have a chronic intestinal inflammation limited to the site of the scar from the operation. Otherwise I am in good shape. Now and then I get arthritic pains in the joints of my right hand when I'm moving, doing push-ups and bench-presses. The tips of my right little finger and ring finger get numb. It has been that way for years. My sugar levels are again quite good and in the normal range. My gastric problem is made worse with gas-producing foods. Where the scar is, there is still inflammation. I had intestinal polyps, which they removed. Possibly for thirty years I have had an ulcerous inflammation there. Ever since dislocating my left shoulder I've had cracking in my left shoulder, and when I play sports there's a drawing pain. In the region of my lumbar spine I get strong pains no matter what the position, first on the right, then the left. Massage, bending over, and warmth all help. After standing a long time I get a drawing pain in my hips. I have mild hip dysplasia on the left side.

Fat foods don't agree with me. I also can't tolerate too many apples, which give me gas. My neck cracks when I twist it. When the weather changes to wet and cold I get drawing pains in my left knee. Earlier my sores would heal almost too fast. In 1983 I was bitten by a mouse and got a rabies injection. At that time I also got a tick-bite.

I become hoarse if I talk a lot. I have nodules on my vocal cords. My blood pressure is normal, even though I stopped taking the tablets. Off and on I get humming in my ears which alternates sides. I always have it when it's quiet. It disturbs my sleep. Now and then it is sometimes gone. Earlier I had gout pains in my big toe. I don't have these anymore. I play a lot of sports. I worry that there will be a recurrence of the Lyme disease.

Analysis: The fact that there is conscious worry about Lyme disease shows that the problem is not yet overcome. However, I was encouraged to include this case here, on account of the relatively long periods that were symptom-free, along with the disappearance of many previous symptoms. When the current Lyme-induced complaints alleviate, then according to natural law older afflictions appear, such as the gastric problems which for the time being intensified, and thus had to be treated homeopathically. That also means that the longer the medical record (many operations, over-drugging, inoculations) the longer the healing will take.

Follow-up/Comment: [April 7, 2004] The gastric complaints have disappeared, but the knee pains have begun again. This case is not over, even with regards to the Lyme condition. However, I have decided to include this account in order to show the kind of detours that we must recognize during homeopathic treatment, when old symptom patterns emerge from the patient's past. Because the life-force was occupying itself with a different chronic disease, these other symptoms had to bide their time under the circumstances. However, these various complaints are mutually dependent and are inseparably connected one with the other. Of course a urologist or an orthopedic surgeon would see things differently, because all such experts are trained only to perceive organs, and not the whole person. Under holistic treatment the patient's own organism determines the direction and pace of healing. We follow in this direction with our remedies, always prepared to supply that organism with the healing stimulus, needed momentarily at that stage of unfolding.

Case 13

Consultation: October 8, 2002
Physician: Peter Alex, Veterinarian and Naturopathic physician, Wildschütz, Germany
Patient: Male, 23 years

Family history:
Ma g'dmother: twin, cardiac infarct at 70
Pa g'father: triplet
Ma g'dfather: cancer of the stomach and eye; 3x cardiac infarcts
Aunt: unstable psychologically

I've had headaches for seven weeks. They began while serving during a church-sponsored retreat as a youth worker abroad. I was vomiting and was nauseous. I couldn't sleep. For a week I've been seeing double at distances of five to one hundred metres. That's quite new. I have pressure bearing down on my ears. The headaches began on the ferry, in the morning when I turned my head. It was as if my brain was loose. It was the first time in my life that I had traveled on a boat. After the trip it became worse while on vacation. At first the headaches were worse with motion, with mental effort as in reading, and with noise (however soft) and bright light. It got so bad that I couldn't sleep at night. On one occasion things improved while playing football. Then the vomiting began nightly. I vomited until noon, after which it was better until evening. Then it got worse after lying down, around two or three in the morning. Suspecting meningitis, they gave me a blood test. They only determined that I had an extremely high leucocyte count. The headaches improve with sleep, and they are generally better since I went to see a chiropractor on account of the vertebrae in my neck. On the journey there, I got chilled, what's more, because of the air conditioning. I came down with a head cold, a teasing cough and a throat inflammation. During my course I slept very little, around five hours a night, for twelve days straight. A computer tomography test showed an arachnoid cyst about 5 x 5 x 3 cm. The headaches are like a pressure on my skull, as if it was inflated, with stabbing pains in my forehead, first to the right, then to the left above the eyes. Mostly I wake around two o'clock and the pains last until dawn. After that I can sleep. Up till noon it was the worst and I threw up, which only worsened the headaches.

[Food?] I eat everything, except I don't like raspberries and blackberries.

[His face is pale and there are red rings beneath his eyes.]

Occasionally my body feels weak and I get dizzy. Sometimes I have spells where I sway from the dizziness. Afterwards the vomiting is worse.

[Tick bites?] In the last five years I've often got bitten, most recently two years ago. About ten years ago I was bitten by a dog. In Greece, I got a lot of mosquito bites. For four days my feet have been permanently cold, which is new. Very hot showers (>40° C.) on my head and neck relieve the headaches, as does a hot towel on my neck or a hot water bottle. In my lumbar spine I have a problem with pinched nerves. I often have had sciatic pains, most recently in 2001 (repeatedly). The pains extend down my right leg.

As a child I stayed awake at night for fear of the dark. I lay wake in the same position in which I lay down. I dreamt that my stuffed animals were attacking me, and I was afraid.

Up until two years ago I was into drugs. For about five years I used cannabis, LSD and psilocybin. At last I had a vision, in which Jesus said, "Decide whether you are for me or against me." In that period I gained a glimpse into the spiritual world, where angels and demons fought each other for each and every person. There were black and white beings. I was very influenced by the black ones, and took the side of evil. I threw away hundreds of dollars on dope yet had no withdrawal symptoms. In the last year a prophetic vision developed, where I bore witness to the end of the world. I felt grief for humanity. I can't alter the course of things, but I am sorry for those who avoid the big picture. I turn towards those who want to make my prophesies known. I am brewing with fresh thoughts, which I believe are sent from God. When I read accounts from other visionaries, I suddenly begin to bawl, because they are so tragic. In church while singing songs of joy I suddenly burst into tears.

Earlier I had fear of high places. Since I took up climbing, that is gone. I am quite gregarious and like to play the leader. I would like to establish what is to be done in a particular situation. If contradicted, I can only accept it if it is on reasonable grounds. Otherwise there are problems. In such situations I say, "Do as you want, but you'll see, it won't work."

As a child I was hyper-active and under-challenged in school. My grades were poor. But to get good results I never had to do a lot. In my opinion I am hard to win over. I am almost never angry. During my school years I had outbursts of anger, but they never achieved their end. I cover up and stayed calm. It is easy for me to assume responsibility. That was there from the beginning. I liked helping people who had lost a relative.

I was vaccinated four times [!] against Russian spring/summer encephalitis, most recently two years ago [German authorities recommend this vaccine as a prophylactic against tick-borne disease, even though only 1 % of all tick-borne disease show an encephalitic profile].

[*Mobile phone or transmission tower in your neighborhood?*] I have a cell-phone and I make a lot of calls with it.

[*Other notable events, especially before the outbreak of symptoms seven or eight weeks ago?*] I feel great sorrow for mankind. That developed strongly during the retreat in Greece. One evening we gave the participants an opportunity to declare themselves for Jesus, to choose the right path, and no one took it. I was shook to the core and severely depressed like never before. I was depressed that I had misled people, as if I am guilty of that. That was two days before I left. I like leading, being a mentor type. I am good at motivating people to develop their capabilities, and I can easily get carried away.

Analysis: With this patient there is a pronounced tendency to share his religious knowledge and experiences with others. For this reason he regards himself as a mentor type (pointing towards a remedy from the gold series.) It was a crushing blow, enough to trigger a Lyme episode, that in spite of his intensive, weeklong efforts during his period of service, no one wanted to profess their beliefs.

The following *MacRepertory* rubrics seem relevant in analyzing the case:

GENERALS, sea-voyage, complaints from — *Arsenicum album* (2)
HEAD, loose, feeling, the brain is — *Arsenicum album* (2)
GENERALS, misuse, drugs, of — *Arsenicum album* (1)
GENERALS, heat aggravates — *Arsenicum album* (1), *Aurum* (2)
MIND, prophesying — *Medorrhinum* (1)
MIND, delusion, he has neglected his duty — *Arsenicum album* (2), *Aurum* (3), *Aurum arsenicosum* (1), *Medorrhinum (1)*
MIND, ailments from anger, vexation — *Aurum* (2)
HEAD, Hair, baldness — *Arsenicum album* (1), *Aurum* (1), *Medorrhinum* (1)
MIND, religious fanaticism — *Aurum arsenicosum* (1), *Medorrhinum* (1)
MIND, feeling of responsibility, over responsible — *Aurum* (1)
MIND, weeping, causeless — *Arsenicum album* (1) *Aurum* (1)
MIND, sadness, music, from — *Arsenicum album* (1)

In analyzing the case, according to Hahnemann's directions only the "characteristic and peculiar ... signs and symptoms" were selected. These are mainly situated in the mental sphere, where the triggering event is highly specific and characteristic. The emergence of *Medorrhinum* during the repertorisation points to a possible taint from the sycotic miasm, which — as I learned in the interval — often underlies Lyme-related illnesses.

Prescription: Aurum arsenicosum LM 12, Dil. 1, 1 x daily, 3 drops

It was further recommended that the patient avoid the use of cell phones and wireless phones using pulsed, high frequency fields. Upon my advice he had a laboratory test done for Lyme disease, which showed up positive.

Follow-up: [November 11, 2002] The headaches and nausea are gone. Overall I feel quite well. Now and then after mental or physical strain I get headaches.

The pains start in my eyes, as if there is increased pressure in the eyeballs, which are actually okay. The tendency to cry has disappeared. I'm back to work full-time. Three times in the interval I've had difficulties with the motor function in my left hand. That hasn't happened for three weeks.

Prescription: Repeat the remedy every two days until the next appointment

Analysis: With this case there is a very short follow-up period, and it is not yet closed. However, it is quite striking how quickly, even in a difficult neurological case, a clear improvement can take place, when the homeopathic simillimum is identified.

Case 14

Consultation: February 2, 2003
Physician: Peter Alex, Veterinarian and Naturopathic physician, Wildschütz, Germany
Patient: Female teacher, 59 years old

Family history:
Mother: depression/ suicide
Gr'father: depression
Uncle: depression
Father: depression and bladder cancer (at 70)

[Grey hair, grey attire.]

I have maddening pains in my right shoulder, which have become better from acupuncture. The right side of my face is paralyzed from an operation in 1987. In August 2001 I got a tick bite on my right leg. It became enormously swollen.

[Her speech is somewhat indistinct due to the facial paralysis.]

Sometimes it's this and sometimes that. A total tiredness and weakness that at times leaves me unable to raise my arms. Sometimes I say to myself, "You're just faking it." In 1987 I had an operation for a neurinoma on my acoustic nerve (causing deafness in the right ear). Since then the right facial nerve is paralyzed and I have problems with my balance. The dizziness is worse since the Lyme disease. I stagger visibly when I walk, worse at twilight. The dizziness is chronic, but worse since the Lyme disease, better sitting and lying, worse on the stairs — then I start swaying with a tendency to fall to the right. I have my reservations about pharmaceutical medicines.

As a child I had measles, mumps, and was quite fit, except I got an inexplicable long-lasting fever. I didn't want to go to school.

I couldn't tolerate Rocephin. I took hormones for my menopausal complaints. Soya hormones helped the climacteric hot flushes. For around one year I have had chronic pain on the left elbow (on the inner condyle), worse from pressure and movement.

[*Joint pains?*] In my knee, sometimes the one, sometimes both. Pressing pain, unaffected by movement, inside the joint. In my shoulders, especially the right, I have chiefly downward pressing pains, such that at times I cannot lie on my right side. For a year now it is sometimes there, sometimes not, coming suddenly and going suddenly, lasting a few minutes to some hours. I have cramp-like pains in my jaw, only in the rigrt lower jaw, radiating to the area of my right collarbone and wandering to my back and chest area. I have wandering pains in my joints. Back pains from scoliosis, chronic pain in the lumbar vertebrae, worse when sitting and getting up, when starting to walk, for around 8 years, worse in the last three years.

[*Sleep?*] For the past year my sleep has been disturbed. I have insomnia until 5 — 5:30 a.m., then I sleep around 2- 3 hours, worse from anticipatory anxiety. I can go to sleep only with heavy sleeping pills, which make the staggering worse. Previously it took an hour for me to go to sleep. I shake in my sleep every few minutes.

[*Dreams?*] Recently I have had nightmares (repeatedly.) I had to climb a church tower, a steep stairway, then the stairs stopped and there were ropes which I was to go up on. A narrow wooden plank over a deep abyss and the banister giving way. I couldn't cross.

I dream of things which I read about during the day. I have absolutely crazy experiences in my dreams.

I did something inappropriate with a little baby.

There are often themes from the previous day, yet absolutely over the top, about something that happens to me, after reading a crime novel. [*laughs nervously*]

At times pressing pains, as if there was air inside my back (already there prior to the Lyme disease), in my stomach like gas which doesn't exit, sometimes for hours.

On the right side of my neck I have a painfully swollen lymph node, even though the nerve is dead. Since my operation every disease lasts longer, colds with chronic run-down state. At work there is always time pressure and deadlines. Since 1985 there has been increasing time pressure, which I find exhausting.

[*What may have triggered the tumor?*] I'm afraid of people (shy). I had to be in front of lots of them.

In 1986 my father died and my mother committed suicide afterwards. I developed guilt feelings. The staggering got worse and the hearing on the right side deteriorated. Occasionally through lack of drive I can sit for hours and do nothing and everything is just too much. The weakness is there upon waking, worse in the morning until around 6 p.m., after which it gets better. I am alone a lot, my husband works in X. I can pull myself together and pretend I was alright. Just let me take my mind off the weakness, especially amongst people. I have suppressed my shyness around people. When I encounter acquaintances, I switch to the other side of the street, from a feeling of inferiority, which my father also used to do. I was never self-conscious, it is somewhat better during work. I have guilt feelings towards others, who could say things behind my back.

I was less shy as a child. I liked doing theater and acting.

[*Aversions?*] Snakes

[*Hobbies?*] Listening to music and singing, gardening, which I am not so bad at. I like unspoilt nature. Reading, strolling, bicycle riding — which I can't do so much, on account of my weakness.

[*Weather?*] Nothing special.

In 1996 I had a uterine prolapse with incontinence. That followed an ovario-hysterectomy, and I have had hot flushes ever since. Despite the medicine they returned and have been worse the last 14 days. The hot flushes with sweat accompany physical effort (the simplest effort such as making breakfast.) My teeth became quite bad after the brain operation. I have a lot of silver, palladium and the like as fillings in my mouth. For the last two years my blood pressure is 160/110.

[*Indigestibles?*] None

[*Aversions?*] None

[*Cravings?*] Milk and carbohydrates.

For around two years I have had diarrhea on occasion, possibly from diverticulitis. I got swollen lymph nodes under my ear from toxoplasmosis in 1978. For 1 to 1-1/2 years I have had spasms at night, lasting around one to two seconds, as if a shudder was passing over my whole body. It is worse especially after going to sleep and before waking up, when they last 9 to 20 seconds — on average 17 seconds, as my husband once calculated. I sleep well during these spasms.

Virological assays from October 25, 2002:

Herpes simplex virus IgG-antibodies	positive
VARICELLA zoster antibody	positive
Epstein-Barr virus antibody	positive

Lab reports from October 19, 2001:

Lyme IgM ELISA	positive
Lyme IgM Western blot	positive

Repertorisation (MacRepertory):

MIND, fear of people — *Arsenicum album* (1), *Aurum* (2)

MIND, speech, abrupt — *Arsenicum album*

EXTREMITIES: Pains, wandering, joints — *Arsenicum album* (2), *Aurum* (3)

HEAD, tumors, brain — *Arsenicum album* (2)

GENERALS, wounds, bites from poisonous animals — *Arsenicum album* (2), *Aurum* (1)

GENERALS, shuddering in sleep — *Arsenicum album* (3)

MIND, gestures while talking — *Arsenicum album* (2)

MIND, cannot bear to be seen — *Arsenicum album* (3)

MIND, delusion, crime, that she is guilty of a crime — *Arsenicum album* (2), *Aurum* (2)

GENERALS, food, craves milk — *Arsenicum album* (2), *Aurum* (1)

SLEEP, sleeplessness, total — *Arsenicum album* (1), *Aurum* (1)

GENERALS, high blood pressure — *Arsenicum album* (1), *Aurum* (2)

Prescription: Aurum arsenicosum LM 30 (ARCANA), 1 x daily, 3 drops

Follow-up: [March 13, 2003] My strength returned and I am on the whole more cheerful. The shoulder pain is gone. The elbows are unchanged, the left being worse. For about three months I occasionally get muscle pains in the right leg, from above to below, while lying down at night [*not mentioned in the initial interview*]. They were worse after *Aurum arsenicosum*, now they are much better, and come at wider intervals. The diarrhea is unchanged, intermittent and alternating with normal stool. Diarrhea 1-2 times a day, and the gurgling in my stomach is more frequent. The hot flushes are more frequent, almost daily. I have no more nightmares. The dizziness, though, is worse. Pain in the lumbar vertebrae on rising from sitting and starting to walk. The cramp-like pain from the right jaw to the clavicle is gone. For around 1 year I have had a constant tingling in my right thigh, manifesting at times as red spots, which are hard to heal. Sometimes itching, which I may or may not scratch. Now I go to sleep around 3 a.m., instead of 5 a.m..

[*High blood pressure?*] I take half a pill.

Prescription: Borrelia MK (Helios). If nothing special happens, begin a week later with *Aurum arsenicosum* LM 45 (ARCANA)

Comment: This prescription was not right on the button, but was more an expression of my indecision. My recommending the *Borrelia* nosode came straight from Ravi Roy via Rocco Kirch. I really didn't want to abandon the remedy that had such a good effect at the outset. Today I would avoid dosing with the nosode, and would even advise against using it at all.

Follow-up: [May 6, 2003] *(As nothing special happened after taking the Borrelia nosode, patient took Aurum arsenicosum LM 45.)* I feel amazingly better, outstanding. The elbow pains are still there a little, but only now and then. Rarely do I have cramping in my right jaw, except during a flu or under stress. Only once did I have pressure in my back as if I was bloated. The itching rash on my thigh is gone. In my lumbar spine there are burning, stitching pains, unconnected to the Lyme disease. I have had scoliosis since my childhood. At times after sitting I cannot get up. It's worse after sitting or standing for a long time, but better after bending over or curling up. While lying I have to keep changing my position. The constant dizziness, which followed the neurinoma operation, has got much less. Ever since the antibiotic treatment in the Autumn of 2001 I have had diarrhea consistently two or three times in the morning, which drives me from the bed. Made worse with Rocephin, before which it was not daily. My stool, which looks bright yellow-orange, squirts out and leaves me sore. It's quite forceful and once it escaped involuntarily. The nightmares are gone. The hot flushes and sweating are much better. The bladder incontinence that comes with motion (which has continued since the operation) is better. The pains in my right leg are better, and the spasms in my sleep have noticeably lessened. From my childhood I have always had stooped shoulders and a rounded back. I sleep well. My blood pressure has been 160/105 for around 2 or 3 years. I never notice it!

[*Dizziness?*] Worse going up stairs and in the twilight.

Prescription: Aurum arsenicosum LM 75 (ARCANA)

Follow-up: [July 2, 2003] My stool is regular and the complaints are almost gone. The dizziness is unchanged, and was even worse after the nosode. On the street I totter. The cramp in my jaw, the pains in my right leg and in my elbow have all completely gone. I have intense pains in the nape of my neck, radiating from the right shoulder blade to my head, which keep me awake until 4 a.m. The pains improve with acupuncture [*old symptom from 14 months ago*]. The aching in my lumbar spine is somewhat better. My sleep was good until the back pains. I was restless and couldn't sleep until 4 a.m. I still jerk in my sleep before waking up. My blood pressure is 161/107. The dizziness is worse at twilight, but normal on the stairs. The dizziness manifests as whirling and as waving lines. I was nauseous for three weeks and my head began feeling heavy from the pains in my neck. The hot flushes are much better and occur only faintly once a day. The vertigo is worse walking backwards, with heavy lifting, bicycle riding and standing on one leg. My bladder incontinence is around 80% better.

Prescription: Aurum arsenicosum MK (Homeoden)

Follow-up: [August 6, 2003] The acupuncture isn't helping so much. I have sharp pains in my neck, which are worse for running and standing around.

After going for a stroll I got burning pains in my hip joint, worse with heat and movement. On occasion I get insomnia, at times bad. For 1-1/2 weeks I have had diarrhea, which is chronic, painless and accompanied by gurgling in my abdomen. I have pressing-drawing pains in my right leg, which ache from the hip downward. The jerking in my sleep has become better. My blood pressure is 149/105. I have had this dizzy feeling ever since the neurinoma operation. The high blood pressure came only later, without symptoms. Taking beta-blockers doesn't make any difference. The CT scan, which the neurologist arranged, came back negative.

Comment: Some symptoms were very much improved under *Aurum arsenicosum*, but others not. This suggests that a further disease, which doesn't have much in common with the first, exists in parallel and must be treated separately. I have frequently noticed this among patients who had undergone brain operations with iatrogenic consequences.

Repertorization:

RECTUM, diarrhea, chronic — *Natrum sulphuricum* (2)

BACK, pain, general, cervical — *Natrum sulphuricum* (2)

HEAD, injury, result of — *Natrum sulphuricum* (3)

DIZZINESS, tendency to fall, to the right — *Natrum sulphuricum (1)*

Prescription: Natrum sulphuricum LM30 (ARCANA)

Follow-up: [October 1, 2003] The cervical pains and the diarrhea are gone. Vertigo unchanged, the pain in my leg and hip is gone. The pains in my lumbar spine are much better; sleep is much better, the joint-pains in my arm and knee have not returned. Since the neurinoma I would fall backwards as soon as I bend my head back. At such times I have to hold onto something. The neurinoma had caused hearing distortions. It was hard to hear on the right, then it gradually went to nothing. I have had hearing problems since 1985. At that time I had quite bad headaches, cutting or sticking in my forehead, several times a week with nausea, so that I had to lie down and close my eyes. These headaches stopped after the tumor operation.

Relations with my parents were stressful. I had an inferiority complex. Then there was a change of director at my work. I was made the acting director, but someone pushed her way forward and took the position away from me.

[*What were the feelings around that?*] I recognized that I was not a director type. However my ambition was awakened. It was a defeat, later I felt it as relief. I have put up with it, I can quickly forget this kind of things — I did my work, she would direct. She had connections everywhere, myself I had none. *Aurum arsenicosum* had improved the hot flashes, which have now returned.

Prescription: *Aurum arsenicosum* MK (Homeoden)

Follow-up: [November 12, 2003] Whatever had returned abruptly went away. The hot flushes are gone. It helped a lot. Can it be that the effect will now slacken off and the condition will return? The archetype of power, which I once felt, is back.

Prescription: 1 globule of *Aurum arsenicosum* MK dissolved in alcohol, and with any return of symptoms, take 1 x 3 drops.

Comment: In contemplating this case one is struck by the complexity of her problems, especially after numerous allopathic therapeutic interventions. For this reason I myself was surprised at the improvements that resulted. This case repeatedly demonstrated how clearly the sycotic miasm emerged from beneath the Lyme disease onto the surface – that is, if one understands *Natrum sulphuricum* as a typical anti-sycotic remedy. In addition, her high blood pressure, which seemed to cause few or no symptoms, is a characteristic of *Aurum arsenicosum*, as I know from other cases.

To this point we have hardly mentioned her high blood pressure and her vertigo, which persisted from the time of the tumor on her auditory nerve. From a therapeutic viewpoint they might need further consideration, but not from the view of the patient herself. As happens so frequently after brain operations, one has to assume that such symptoms will never go away, for when the cerebral nerves are damaged, they are not capable of regeneration.

2-1/2 years following our last consultation I asked her permission to publish the case, and she told me that since that time she had maintained good health, although she had had to repeat the remedy a few times.

Follow-up: [May 18 2006] Part of her symptoms came back, such as sleeplessness, depression, hip pain, pain in her lower back on rising from a chair and a weakness in her legs.

First I tried *Aurum arsenicosum* XMK, which according to my clinical experiences, should afford prompt relief if it was a relapse of the Lyme disease. In her case it did not do anything within 2 weeks, so I looked at her case again and found the following characteristics:

MIND, Indifference towards pleasure — *Agar.* (1)

HEAD, cerebral hemorrhage (as a result of her brain tumor operation) — *Agar.* (1)

SPEECH, jerks, by — *Agar.* (1)

BACK, pain, general, lumbar, rising from sitting — *Agar.* (3)

EXTREMITIES, pain, hip, extending down leg — *Agar.* (2)

EXTREMITIES, weakness, leg — *Agar.* (1)

SLEEP, sleeplessness, after midnight, after 4 a.m. — *Agar. (2)*

Prescription: *Agaricus muscarius* Q 2 (Gudjons), 2 drops daily

Follow-up: [June 8, 2006] My sleep is all right. The pain in my hip and leg was gone most days. The depression and low feeling has not changed despite my sleeping much better.

Comment: The course of homeopathic treatment has to follow the medical biography of the patient, only in reverse. After we overcame the tick-caused disease (*Aurum arsenicosum*), we had to deal with the after- effects of her brain operation (*Natrum sulphuricum* and *Agaricus muscarius*). Now we see her depression as the only remaining and so far deepest discernible layer (see family anamnesis!) of disease in this patient. For any one familiar with Hering's law this pattern had to emerge sometime and will have to be taken care of homeopathically. This case is an example of several dissimilar diseases existing in one person, which — as Hahnemann mentions in the *Organon* — have to be treated in sequence.

Case 15

Consultation:	June 15, 2004
Doctor:	Peter Alex, Veterinarian and Naturopathic physician, Wildschuetz, Germany
Patient:	A 69-year-old pensioner, a doctor of engineering science, who was in my care from 1996-1999 for a fungal infection of his nails
Family:	cancer, TB, manic-depressive, diabetes I, many stomach ulcers both on the mother's and father's side, alcoholism.

Note: The patient was treated anti-miasmatically by a very experienced homeopath. From September 1999 to April 2004 she prescribed the following remedies, which the patient meticulously recorded: *X-ray; Mercurius* 200C; *Nitricum acidum* LM 6, 12, 18; *Arsenicum album* LM 6, 18, 24, 45, 60 (which improved the fungus infection); *Veratrum album* 30C; *Sulphur* 30C; *Colocynthis* LM6 (which caused a remedy proving); *Mercurius vivus* (after tick bites); *Thuja* 200C; *Staphysagria* LM12; *Lycopodium* LM 6; Thuja LM 6, 12, 18, 24 (which caused his hands to tremble); *Borrelia* nosode LM 12, 18; *Mercurius* LM 24.

... Since my 40th year I've had aching pains in my knees. In 2001 they were almost gone, but after July 2003 they came back, following a tick bite. In November 2003 my knee pains started up again on the left side. The pains are worse with stretching (the leg can't stretch out) and also with bending the leg. Cooling improves the situation. Previously I was into athletics on a competitive basis. Since April 2004 there has been pain in my right knee on the medial tibial head. The knee-pains used to begin when I was visiting an exhibition. The pains are always aching. I can't kneel down. The knee hurts while I'm walking. I had an operation for a ganglion in the hollow of my right knee.

The place where the tick bit still has a lilac colour and is about the diameter of a 5-cent piece. Recently it suppurated. Afterwards I went on an alpine tour: The wound-site hurt and the redness traveled up to my chest and left arm. I got antibiotics. I have had reduced colour vision ever since a scarlet- fever infection in my youth. I've had this fungal infection on my nails intermittently since 1994. It came and went under homeopathic treatment. Now it's definitely in remission.

I suffered from depression. After my daughter had her fourth child, because we didn't have our own suite, the house became too small for us grandparents. We uprooted and bought a new house in the country. That caused a lot of problems for me, for the house was my life's work, I still haven't learned to cope. I suffer from feelings of betrayal. Previously we made decisions together (at the time of the first child). It wounded my feelings. Perhaps we expected too much? We were a bit angry. I was isolated from my previous round of activities. I asked myself if I did the right thing. There's some restlessness in me, and without a car we were as good as dead out there [at the new place, 40 km from the city]. I think a lot about the future. From a skiing accident in February 2003 I dislocated my upper right shoulder – and not for the first time. I take everything too seriously. I can lose myself in trivialities — but I also have a good outlook. Inwardly I resisted moving to another place.

After the tick-bite I got a rough swelling on my thigh, which lasted a year. After a tick bite in 1998 I got bad knee pains and my cervical spine tensed up. After taking antibiotics I got ear problems.

Cannot tolerate: food and drink at refrigerator temperatures
Desires: sweet, very spicy, fish
Avoids: ice-cream, fatty beef, sour fruit

Usually my stool was unformed; now it has been firm for some time. I tend to have cold feet and hands. I feel worse when I watch TV (no matter what), which I find amusing. At times all of a sudden I get a "sneezing fit" with my eyes "watering buckets." I live only 300 metres from the [wireless phone] radio antenna. [*This helped confirm my suspicion that there is a link between the sensitivity to or impairment from cell-phones and the susceptibility to Lyme disease.*] For decades I have got up early and slept poorly. At times I feel as if I haven't slept at all. I feel that things come up which take the form of dreams, but these I can hardly remember. For example, they resolve problems that arise. About once or twice a week I have a nocturnal urge to urinate. I wake in a great heat (have to get out of my pyjamas, though I really enjoy warmth.) I wake from my sleep around 2:30 to 4 a.m., and then I doze until the early dawn, snoring a little. I was never a memory prodigy, and my memory for names has become worse.

Task solutions come to me in dreams, the catch being to record them. I go to sleep easily, as long as I don't think about things.

[*Psychological condition*] During the purchase of our house I didn't want to see the notary, but wanted to run away instead. I was temporarily lethargic, which usually isn't my style, to the point that I became suicidal. Recently I have had financial worries on account of my loan. The urge to urinate is somewhat worse. I get drawing pains on the sole of my right heel, after hiking for a time. They reach to my shin. My knee hurts when I cross my legs. During long automobile rides I feel a tension in my shoulder and neck area. It has improved since taking Bowen therapy. For a long time I have done alpine hiking. Last year I went back to climbing. I didn't know the safety procedures any more. and I asked myself, "Will I make a fool of myself, because I no longer have what it takes?" I wasn't used to dealing with that type of rock. The distal joint of my left thumb has been hurting for about a year from bending or heavy pressure. In 2003 I had drawing heart pain and the sense of an elevated pulse in the morning upon waking. Once a day in 2003 I had prolonged, intense headaches, which I never had before.

[*Do you have depressive times?*] I spent two months in Spain. After my return I got it again. At such times I tend just to lie in bed, with no drive, although I am usually active. I didn't want to be uprooted. It's a stupid thing to get old there. I feel like I am a kind of hybrid. I have never been part of a choir, but now I've joined one. If I can get a foothold here, then I have arrived. I thought it might pass.

I like going to concerts or the church. My problem is homesickness. I like being by the water, in the mountains; I love the ever-changing landscape, the flowering meadows, paddling and camping in the wild. All my life I was singled out by stinging insects! Perhaps I have to consider being less active. I have a desire to travel. In June 2002 I was vaccinated against the flu.

Prescription: *Ignatia* MK (for what I thought was the acute condition)

Follow-up: My knee hurts more when I'm walking slowly than when I'm running fast. The finger joints are unchanged. After taking *Ignatia* I felt a pain in the opposite side, where the tick bite was! The day before yesterday

I had "head pains," a slight aching on the left side [*old symptom*]. I still can't sleep from 3:30 to 5 a.m. Like Mephisto's alter ego, my critical side gains the upper hand. Whenever I mull over something that permits of innovation, I know what to do as soon as I wake up. I had a depressive phase (before taking the remedy) that was linked to my change of residence. Whenever I became listless, I told myself forcefully, "You must!" I was not communicative, but inwardly felt rage, which I turned on myself. I am critical and angry about my mistakes. Stomach problems start up after a conversation [*prior to taking the remedy*]. I get a loud gurgling in my belly, with drawing pains in my stomach. These are worse after eating bloating food. I have halitosis. Frequently I have the urge to pass stool without doing so. I am better with classical music (church music). The heel pain is unchanged.

Analysis: Although the patient had been treated by an experienced homeopath for his inherited weaknesses (miasms), his Lyme-related complaints did not improve at all. My colleague was so in despair over this, that she advised him to take antibiotic treatment. After I had eliminated the acute trouble as an obstacle to health (the dose of *Ignatia*), I resolved to try *Aurum arsenicosum*, which I had in the meantime frequently extolled as the "Lyme remedy." After all, if not his very appearance, then many things in the case history point to this remedy.

Repertory rubrics:

MIND, memory, weakness, loss of, for names — *Aurum* (1)

MIND, ailments from mortification, humiliation, chagrin — *Arsenicum album* (2), *Aurum* (2)

MIND, conscientious about trifles — *Arsenicum album* (4), *Aurum* (1)

MIND, fear of poverty, anxiety about business — *Arsenicum album* (1) *Aurum* (1)

MIND, music ameliorates, classical music — *Aurum* (2)

GENERALS, pains in the limbs, lower limbs, knee, while walking — *Aurum* (2)

SLEEP, waking, from and with heat — *Arsenicum album* (1)

SLEEP, sleepless from 2-4 a.m. — *Arsenicum album* (3), *Aurum* (1)

RECTUM, diarrhea, general, elderly people — *Arsenicum album* (3)

Prescription: Aurum arsenicosum 200C

Follow-up: [August 17, 2004] My overall state is great so far. Even on a 700- meter climb in the Alps I had no knee complaints. I still have pain remaining in my abdomen, but even that is better. I began jogging four weeks ago. I climbed over 4,000 meters and descended 4,000 on the Ortler [*one of the highest mountains in the Alps*]. My sleep continued improving. Every second day I couldn't sleep after 5 a.m. A pustule appeared on the left middle finger, which lasted a week. The site of the tick bite is still rose-coloured. My memory for information has deteriorated. I forget the names for mountains, cable railways, and so on.

I had more than ten tick bites! I don't go to the bathroom so frequently, have no diarrhea, and can tolerate coffee! I was in a blessed state of mind after climbing the glacier at 3,300 meters. That was a miracle, for I didn't want to trek in the mountains on account of the pains in my heel — of which only a little remains. I can't stretch out my knee entirely — there is still a "threshold pain" there.

Prescription: Aurum arsenicosum MK

Follow-up: [October 2004, via phone] My joint ailments keep improving. My overall state of health is very good.

Comment: This case may serve as evidence that *Aurum arsenicosum* can be a remedy in the healing of the Lyme miasm (if one chooses thus to label a chronic weakness acquired from that infection.) The patient is still under my treatment. The joint pains returned in summer 2005 and subsided completely up to this point [June 2006] after another dose of *Aurum arsenicosum* MK. He continues roaming the world without physical limitations.

Despite the complete remission of Lyme-related symptoms the lab test still shows a raised antibody-titer. The titer went from 140 units/ml in May 2004 down to 110 units/ml in March 2005 (when the last test was done). Could it be that the reduction of antibody titer is slower in elderly patients? Ordinarily I have seen the antibody titer return to normal within 6 months after the symptoms have disappeared. This is a treatment variable that requires further research.

As in the case with about 50 % of my Lyme patients, in this patient a *Medorrhinum* picture now emerged:

MIND, memory, weakness, names, for proper — *Med.* (2)

HEAD, pain, exposure to sun, from — *Med.* (1)

CHEST, Pain, heart, extending to left arm — *Med.* (2) [a rarely appearing symptom that he used to have intermittently over a long period, after exerting his shoulder, now returning more strongly]

EXTREMITIES, PAIN, upper limbs, shoulder right — *Med.* (1) [an old symptom that he had for many years after exerting his shoulder, now returned more strongly]

EXTREMITIES, callosities, foot, soles — *Med.* (1)

SLEEP, waking, as if having slept one's fill — *Med.* (1)

Prescription: *Medorrhinum* MK.

Last Follow-up: [June 20, 2006] The shoulder pain that bothered me for several months is gone completely.

Homeopathic Cure of Lyme Disease in Animals

Back in 1994 Stephen Tobin, a Connecticut veterinarian who is versed in holistic medicine, surprised the American public with a magazine article in which he reported having either cured or distinctly improved hundreds of Lyme cases amongst dogs, cats and horses, merely through the use of the remedy *Ledum palustre* 1M, 3 times daily for three days. Although, as noted above, *Ledum* is certainly the remedy of choice in many cases of Lyme arthritis, from our own experiences we have to question this report. In Germany we possibly face a different situation (various Lyme strains, different vectors), which doesn't permit such a drastically simplified procedure. On the other hand, in his publication Tobin does not describe exactly what he means by "an amelioration."

Especially in chronic Lyme cases animals also require an individualizing approach, which homeopathic treatment provides.

Case 16

Consultation:	August 2, 2002
Veterinarian:	Jens Kirchner, Veterinarian and Naturopathic physician, Neubrandenburg, Germany
Patient:	German wire-haired cross, born May, 2001

The dog suddenly displayed extreme lameness in the left rear leg. He was completely wiped out, didn't want to move at all, ate nothing and drank very little. His temperature read 40.1 C. The tarsal joint was warm and clearly swollen. >From March to July, 2002, the dog had between five to 10 ticks every day, which were removed at the time by hand. Fourteen days ago a tick bite became inflamed, but healed over again by itself. While the suspicion about Lyme disease was never far away, it was not confirmed through a titer assay.

As a first remedy I gave the dog *Apis* 30C, 3 x at three hour intervals, but without any reaction. On the basis of his case history the dog then got *Ledum* 200C, one dose of two globules.

His general condition improved so quickly that after one hour he turned cheerful, drank and ate. His temperature fell by two degree into the normal range for a dog. The leg, however, was still not used. I prescribed *Ledum*

6C, five globules, once a day for the next five days. After five days he was using the leg as normal in slower movement, yet continued to favor it when running fast. No further remedy was provided, and around fourteen days after the 200C dose, the dog was able to move in a completely normal way.

It is interesting to note that five weeks after the dose of *Ledum*, the dog didn't pick up one single tick, in spite of the fact that he was back on his own terrain.

Note by Peter Alex:

The critical reader might object that one can't speak here of a Lyme case, since no diagnostic proof was forthcoming from the laboratory. However, we know, being familiar with the literature, that in at least 50% of all cases of acute canine arthritis, a borreliosis can be confirmed. This figure does not include the frequent false negatives that occur with the most widely used (but nevertheless not very reliable) ELISA test. Since animal owners, other than those covered by health insurance, must themselves pay for the full range of veterinary services, practitioners oftentimes dispense with this measure. As much as with allopathic treatment (where NSAI or cortisone are routinely prescribed for symptomatic arthritis), so also in homeopathy (where individual case-taking supplants clinical diagnosis) — in neither case do laboratory results have a role to play therapeutically. For most animal owners it would be indeed hard to justify such a capital-intensive diagnostic.

For our purposes this case serves quite well. It concerns a Lyme-type case of canine arthritis following multiple tick bites, which was healed using a Lyme-appropriate remedy (*Ledum*) in a typical homeopathic fashion — rapid, gentle, safe and permanent.

BIBLIOGRAPHY

Alex, Peter.

2003. Similarity, Analogy and Simultaneity; in Friedrich Wiest and Matthias Varga von Kibed, eds, *The Field of Similars*. Heidelberg: Carl-Auer.

2003. Tetanus; in *Nature & Healing*.

2005. *Heilung Borreliosekranker mit Homoopathie*. Grimma: Edition Krannich.

Barthel, Horst

1995. *Homeopathic Prophylaxis. German Journal of Homeopathy* 1. Berg am Starnberger See: Barthel & Barthel.

Bransfield, R.

Website. The neuropsychiatric assessment of Lyme disease. www.mentalhealthandillness.com

Buchwald, Gerhard

2000. *Vaccination — The Link with Anxiety*. Munich: Knaur.

Burkhardt, Friedrich

1992. *Microbiological Diagnosis*. Stuttgart, New York: Thieme.

Fallon, B.A.

Website. Late-stage neuropsychiatric Lyme borreliosis, differential diagnosis and treatment. www.wadhurst.demon.co.uk.

Fallon, B.A. et al.

Website. The neuropsychiatric manifestations of Lyme borreliosis. www.LymeNet.org

Fine, Howard

1994. Trigeminal neuralgia and palpitation from Lyme disease. *New England Journal of Homeopathy* 1.

Fust, Elfie

1999. *Tick Bites — Disease Pictures and Treatment Possibilities*. Vienna: HF.

Goldings, A.S.

Website. Controversies in neuroborreliosis. www.Ilads.org

Graf, Friedrich
1997. Lecture. The First International Homeopathic Congress on Chronic Diseases. Berlin.

Gray, Bill
1994. *Ledum palustre*. The Homeopath 52.

Grier, T.M.
Website. The complexities of Lyme disease. www.canlyme.com.

Hahnemann, Samuel
1842/1985. *Organon of the Medical Art. 6th Edition*. Berg am Starnberger See: O.-Verlag.
1830-3/1979. *Materia Medica Pura*, vol. 1. Heidelberg: Karl F. Haug.

Heidemann, Horst
Personal communication.

Killian, Vera
1994. Lyme Disease. *Journal of Homeopathy* 2.

Kirch, Rocco
1997. Homeopathic Therapy and Prevention for Insect Stings and Bites. *Homeopathic Guide 16/17* — Man and Beast. Murnau: Lage & Roy.

Krafeld, Karl and Stefan Lanka
2002. *Vaccination — Mass Murder in the Third Millennium?* Eichst tt: Pirol.

Lang, Denise
2004. *Coping with Lyme disease*. New York: Henry Hold & Company

Margulis, Lynn and Dorion Sagan
1991. *Microcosmos: four billion years of evolution from our microbial ancestors*. New York: Simon & Schuster.

Melhorn, Wolf-Alexander
2002. www.melhorn.de/Borreliose/index.htm.

Murphy, Robin
1993. *Homeopathic Medical Repertory*. New Delhi: Indian Books & Periodicals.

Peters, Juergen, ed.
2002. *Lyme Newsletter* 6. Hamburg.

Pietrucha, D.M.
Website. Neurological manifestations of Lyme disease in children. www.Lymealliance.org.

Pitcairn, Richard
1995. A New Look at the Vaccine Question. *Homeopathic Links* 2.

Psychyrembel
1994. *Clinical Dictionary.* Berlin, New York: Walter de Gruyter.

Purkert, Peter
1994. Lyme Disease Often Manifests in Veiled and Subtle Ways. *Journal of Homeopathy* 2.

Riefer, Marco W.
1996. *The Remedy Picture of Candida albicans.* Freiburg: Self-published.

Rissenberg, Marian and Susan Chambers
1998. Distinct pattern of cognitive impairment noted in study of Lyme patients. *Lyme Times* 20, January-March.

Rolle, M. and A. Mayr
Medical Microbiology and Epidemic Research. 7th Edition. Stuttgart: Enke.

Rotundo, Beth
1994. Lyme with the desire to kill. *New England Journal of Homeopathy* 1.

Roy, Ravi and Carola Roy
1993 — 2000. *Homeopathic Guide; The Homeopathic Vaccination; Vaccination; Homeopathic First Aid.* Murnau: Lage & Roy.

Rubel, Joanne
Website. Lyme disease, symptoms & charcteristics: a compilation of peer-reviewed literature reports. www.canlyme.com

Scholten, Jan
1996. *Homeopathy and the Elements.* Utrecht: Alonnissos.

Schuster, Bernd
1994. The Microbe as a Causative Agent. *Homöopathiezeitschrift* 2.

Seiler, Hanspeter
1988. *The Development of Samuel Hahnemann's Medical Practice.* Heidelberg: Karl F. Haug.

Sheldrake, Rupert

2000. *The Memory of Nature*. Munich: Scherz.

Sherr, V.T.

Website. The physician as patient: Lyme disease, ehrlichiosis and babesiosis: a recounting of a personal experience with tick-borne diseases. www.ilads.org.

Splittstoesser, Wulf

1998. *Gold Fever.* Kelkheim: Eigenverlag.

Vermeulen, Frans

1996. *Synoptic Materia Medica*. Two volumes. Haarlem: Marlijn.

2005. *Monera*. Lecture presented at the International Homeopathy Seminar at Den Haag.

Vithoulkas, George

1979. *Medicine of the Future*. Kassel: G. Wenderoth.

Warkentin, David Kent

2000. MacRepertory 5.6: Repertorisation Software. Kent Homeopathic Associates.

Wormser, Gary P. et al.

2000. Practical Guidelines for the Treatment of Lyme Disease. *Clinical Infectious Diseases* 31.

Wulfsberg, Terje

1998. *Three Pieces of Gold*. Oslo: Homeopati Bokhandelen.

Zandvoort, Roger van

2000. Complete Repertory. Leidschendam: IRHIS.